Professional and Practice-based Learning

Volume 7

For further volumes:
http://www.springer.com/series/8383

Series Editors:

Stephen Billett, Griffith University, Australia
Christian Harteis, Paderborn University, Germany
Hans Gruber, University of Regensburg, Germany

Professional and practice-based learning brings together international research on the individual development of professionals and the organisation of professional life and educational experiences. It complements the Springer journal *Vocations and Learning: Studies in vocational and professional education.*

Professional learning, and the practice-based processes that often support it, are the subject of increased interest and attention in the fields of educational, psychological, sociological, and business management research, and also by governments, employer organisations and unions. This professional learning goes beyond, what is often termed professional education, as it includes learning processes and experiences outside of educational institutions in both the initial and ongoing learning for the professional practice. Changes in these workplaces requirements usually manifest themselves in the everyday work tasks, professional development provisions in educational institution decrease in their salience, and learning and development during professional activities increase in their salience.

There are a range of scientific challenges and important focuses within the field of professional learning. These include:

- understanding and making explicit the complex and massive knowledge that is required for professional practice and identifying ways in which this knowledge can best be initially learnt and developed further throughout professional life.
- analytical explications of those processes that support learning at an individual and an organisational level.
- understanding how learning experiences and educational processes might best be aligned or integrated to support professional learning.

The series integrates research from different disciplines: education, sociology, psychology, amongst others. The series is comprehensive in scope as it not only focusses on professional learning of teachers and those in schools, colleges and universities, but all professional development within organisations.

Stephen Billett · Amanda Henderson
Editors

Developing Learning Professionals

Integrating Experiences in University
and Practice Settings

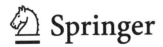 Springer

Editors
Stephen Billett
Griffith University
School of Education &
    Professional Studi
Mount Gravatt Campus
4112 Griffith Queensland
Australia
s.billett@griffith.edu.au

Dr. Amanda Henderson
Queensland Health
Queensland
Australia
and
School of Nursing and Midwifery
Griffith University
Queensland
Australia
Amanda_Henderson@health.qld.gov.au

ISSN 2210-5549
ISBN 978-90-481-3936-1
DOI 10.1007/978-90-481-3937-8
Springer Dordrecht Heidelberg London New York

e-ISSN 2210-5557
e-ISBN 978-90-481-3937-8

Library of Congress Control Number: 2011920831

Printed on acid-free paper

Springer is part of Springer Science+Business Media (www.springer.com)

Series Editors' Foreword

Promoting professional learning has become of increasing interest in many countries because of the growing percentage of professional workers in the workforce, the need to prepare them adequately for their important workplace roles and also to sustain their occupational competence across their working lives. Certainly, much of this interest resides in higher education institutions as they work to fulfil their roles in preparing professionals through their undergraduate and postgraduate programmes. Increasingly, that interest is also being exercised in programmes associated with professional development (i.e. further development of occupational knowledge across working life). One feature of this interest in both of these kinds of educational programmes is how to most effectively utilise and integrate students' experiences in practice settings. That is integrating workplace experiences within the higher education curriculum. Of course, many programmes such as medicine, nursing and education have long utilised, and possibly sought to integrate experiences from practice settings. Practicums, placements and clinical practice have long been elements of programmes in these fields. However, now in both initial preparatory and ongoing developmental programmes, there is growing requirement for not only experiences in appropriate practice setting, but also their effective integration into the course curriculum. Hence, there is need for concepts, models and practices that can inform the implementation of educational process far more widely than in medicine, nursing and teacher education. Therefore, it is timely that this edited monograph is able to illuminate and support discussions about the educational purposes, worth and practices associated with this educational process are made available here.

In overview, this book identifies, discusses and elaborates processes through which professional learning can be effectively promoted through the integration of learning experiences across university and practice settings. Increasingly, programmes in universities from which the studies such as those included in this text are drawn have expectations that graduates will enjoy smooth transitions into professional practice. Hence, the emphasis on work-integrated learning within the higher education programmes, albeit with approaches to provide and integrate experiences in practice settings taking particular forms across the different disciplines. So, offered here are a range of Australian higher education perspectives drawn from a series of nationally funded projects that have investigated processes through which these integrations might proceed. The contributions are drawn from projects that sought to identify the scope and bases for advancing work-integrated learning across the higher education system nationally and those that investigated curriculum and pedagogic practices to support that integration. Collectively, what is advanced through these contributions comprises the findings and synthesis of a series of projects that are seeking to inform the significance of integrating experiences in practice and academic settings. Given the interest, internationally, within higher education to utilise and effectively integrate into higher education curriculum experiences from practice settings, this book should attract a wide readership. Its strengths will be found in its conceptual premises, elaborations and synthesis, the use of actual incidents of practice to elaborate these premises and advance curriculum and pedagogic practices from a range of areas of professional practice.

The contributions of this book focus on the kinds of experiences that can best assist the effective initial preparation of professional practitioners, including a smooth transition into practice and the development of 'learning professionals.' The contributions are provided across three sections. First, the introductory sections set out the procedural and conceptual terrain. This section includes discussions about the worth of the integrations and offers some conceptual bases to assist understand what they comprise and how they need to be ordered as intentional learning experiences. Following this in the section entitled – *Integrating Practice and University Experiences: Curriculum and Pedagogy Practices* – are a set of discipline specific cases from nursing, physiotherapy, midwifery, social work and medicine, including an interdisciplinary study involving medical and nursing students. Each of these chapters reports on distinct kinds of pedagogic and curriculum practices that aim to integrate students experiences for different purposes. Then, and third, in the section entitled – *Institutional Practices and Imperatives* – are contributions that elaborate how career education can be realised through such integrations, how institutions might be best organised to secure such integrations, the ordering of experiences in multidisciplinary work teams in clinical settings. In all, provided here is a text that seeks to elaborate concepts and practices associated with professional and practice-based learning.

(October 2010)

Hans Gruber
Christian Harteis
Stephen Billett

Preface

In countries with both emerging and advanced industrial economies, there are new educational challenges arising from demands for universities and other educational institutions to prepare their students for specific occupations and to be ready to practice in the particular instances of that occupational practice. That is, they are required to be 'job-ready' on graduation. This is an extremely tough educational goal premised upon societal expectations that are not easy to achieve. Yet, this goal would likely be seen by the majority of educators as being the very kind of outcome that they intend for their students. Consequently, not only are parties external to higher education concerned with this kind of goal, but also many, and perhaps most, of those who work in higher and tertiary education are concerned to secure positive and productive learning outcomes for their students. Yet, achieving this educational goal requires the development of the conceptual, procedural and dispositional knowledge needed for competent occupational practice, including the variations of that knowledge necessary to address the specific requirements of particular instances of professional practice in which graduates are employed. In many ways, this challenge is greater than the expectations of schooling, given the specific requirements of particular practice circumstances. Here, there is an imperative for the development of the canonical knowledge of the professions to be learnt robustly and also in ways that make it adaptable to the kinds of practices that graduates will encounter during their courses and directly upon graduation, many of which may be unknown to both the teacher and the student. In addition, there are other goals that, although included within the development of occupational knowledge, may need specific educational considerations. One of these is preparing students to be proactive and self-directed in their occupational practice. A key quality of professionals is for them to be self-monitoring of their practice and self-directing in their ongoing learning. Yet, these capacities will likely need to be developed; they will not necessarily simply arise through students' participation in an educational programme. Moreover, these capacities need to have a contextual dimension because abstract or dis-embedded capacities are unlikely to be helpful in situations that have specific requirements and generate particular kinds of problems.

It is for these reasons that there is a growing imperative in many countries and across a growing range of occupational disciplines not only for graduates to have practice-based experiences throughout their programmes of study, but importantly for these experiences to be integrated within the academic curriculum. More than being merely opportunities to practice and apply what has been learnt in university settings, experiences in practice settings stand as essential learning opportunities in their own right and need to be positioned effectively within the overall curriculum to strengthen and augment what is learnt through taught experiences in educational institutions. That is, they are central to the development of the kinds of knowledge required for effective practice, and also the capacities that will serve graduates well in monitoring and sustaining their effectiveness as occupational practitioners. It follows then that the focus of this volume reflects such imperatives, needs and concerns. The studies discussed within this volume provide distinct accounts of how the development and integration of these experiences can progress to promote professional learning. The contributions findings of several distinct studies are highlighted, and included for understanding the pedagogic, curriculum and institutional bases for professional development. In addition, considerations of appropriate conceptual premises and procedural approaches are used to inform and guide the discussions across these chapters.

Support for this book has been provided by the Australian Learning and Teaching Council Limited, an initiative of the Australian Government Department of Education, Employment and Workplace Relations, and also the Australian Research Council. The views expressed in this book do not necessarily reflect the views of the Australian Learning and Teaching Council, or the Australian Research Council.

It is also important to acknowledge the support of the Griffith Institute for Educational Research in production of this book, most especially the skills and commitment of Ms Andrea Kittila whose editing and formatting work was greatly appreciated by all contributors and the two editors.

Brisbane, QLD   Stephen Billett
Brisbane, QLD   Amanda Henderson
(July 2010)

Series Introduction

This series of books for Springer constitutes an important international forum for studies of professional and practice-based learning. Its origins are located in the need for a focused and cross-disciplinary scholarly forum to propose, explain and further elaborate how learning through and for occupational practice proceeds and how that learning can be promoted and supported. The need for effective occupational preparation is well understood, but increasingly is being extended to practice-based experiences, and their integration within programmes of initial occupational preparation. However, the need for professional learning throughout working lives has become essential within the last decades as the requirements for occupational practices constantly change, and likely become more demanding. Additionally, professional learning is not only a matter of working life, but also a matter of social participation, as successful accomplishment of occupational challenges provides the basis for access to societal resources. In all, occupational development, transitions in individuals' occupational careers, as well as shifts in jobs, activities and tasks make learning throughout working life essential. Also, because changes in these workplace requirements usually manifest themselves in the everyday work tasks, professional development provisions in educational institutions decrease in their salience, and learning and development during professional activities increase in their salience. Consequently, educational enquiry has now to focus on the analysis and the support of learning within and throughout professional life. Scholarship on professional and practice-based learning is, therefore, emerging as a crucial topic within educational enquiry.

Indeed, there is wide interest in such a forum. Professional learning and the practice-based processes that often support it are the subject of great interest and attention in the fields of educational, psychological, sociological and business management research, and also from governments, employer organisations, professional associations and unions. Importantly, the concept of professional learning encompassed in this series goes beyond what is often termed professional education. Instead, it includes learning processes and experiences outside of educational institutions in both the initial and ongoing learning for the professional practice.

Readers can draw on contributions from a range of disciplines and subdisciplinary fields, as they confront a range of scientific challenges and important focuses within the field of professional learning. These include understanding and making explicit the complex and massive knowledge that is required for professional practice and identifying ways in which this knowledge can best be initially learnt and developed further throughout professional life. A major issue of the book series will be analytical explications of those processes that support individuals' learning as well as organisational change.

In all, the series aims to establish itself as a strong and highly esteemed platform for the discussion of concepts of professional learning that focuses on both the individual development of professionals and the organisation of professional life and educational experiences to support and sustain that learning. The series aims to overcome the compartmentalisation of research methods and paradigms by being inclusive of the approaches used in the field of professional and practice-based learning.

Stephen Billett
Hans Gruber
Christian Harteis

Contents

Part II   Institutional Practices and Imperatives

Contributors

Heather Alexander Australian Medical Council, Canberra, Australia,
heathera@amc.org.au

Stephen Billett School of Education and Professional Studies, Griffith University,
Brisbane, QLD 4112, Australia, s.billett@griffith.edu.au

Sally Brooks RMIT University, Melbourne, VIC, Australia,
sally.brooks@rmit.edu.au

Jennifer Cartmel Griffith University, Brisbane, QLD, Australia,
j.cartmel@griffith.edu.au

Natalie Gamble Queensland University of Technology, Brisbane, QLD,
Australia, natalie.gamble@qut.edu.au

Pauline Glover Flinders University, Adelaide, SA 5042, Australia,
pauline.glover@flinders.edu.au

Amanda Henderson Queensland Health, Queensland, Australia; School of
Nursing and Midwifery, Griffith University, Queensland, Australia,
Amanda_Henderson@health.qld.gov.au

Brian Jolly Monash University, Melbourne, VIC, Australia,
brian.jolly@monash.edu

Jenny Keating Monash University, Melbourne, VIC, Australia,
Jenny.Keating@monash.edu

Anna Lichtenberg University of Wollongong, Wollogong, NSW, Australia,
alichtenberg@nd.edu.au

Sue McAllister Flinders University, Adelaide, SA, Australia,
sue.mcallister@flinders.edu.au

Peter McIlveen University of Southern Queensland, Toowoomba, QLD,
Australia, peter.mcilveen@usq.edu.au

Elizabeth Molloy Monash University, Melbourne, VIC, Australia, Elizabeth.Molloy@monash.edu

Jennifer M. Newton School of Nursing and Midwifery, Monash University, Melbourne, VIC, Australia, jenny.newton@monash.edu

Cherene Ockerby Southern Health, Clayton, VIC, Australia, cherene.ockerby@southernhealth.org.au

Maree O'Keefe University of Adelaide, Adelaide, SA, Australia, maree.okeefe@adelaide.edu.au

Deborah Peach Queensland University of Technology, Brisbane, QLD, Australia, d.peach@qut.edu.au

Martin Smith University of Wollongong, Wollogong, NSW, Australia, martin@uow.edu.au

Ieva Stupans University of South Australia, Adelaide, SA, Australia, Ieva.Stupans@unisa.edu.au

Linda Sweet Flinders University, Adelaide, SA 5042, Australia, linda.sweet@flinders.edu.au

Peter Torjul Flinders University, Adelaide, SA, Australia, peter.torjul@flinders.edu.au

Joanne Tyler Monash University, Melbourne, VIC, Australia, joanne.tyler@adm.monash.edu.au

About the Authors

Heather Alexander (Australian Medical Council, Australia) Dr Alexander has a long experience in health professional education, primarily as a medical educator over the last decade and previously as a clinical dietician/nutritionist. She is currently working with the Australian Medical Council overseeing the accreditation process for the implementation of workplace-based assessment for international medical graduates seeking general registration in Australia. She currently holds an adjunct appointment with the Griffith Institute for Higher Education. Her expertise focuses on assessment, including clinical and workplace-based assessment. She was awarded an Associate Fellowship in 2007 by the Australian Learning and Teaching Council for a project establishing interprofessional learning for nursing and medical students while in the clinical setting.

Stephen Billett (Griffith University, Australia) Professor Stephen Billett has worked as a vocational educator, educational administrator, and teacher educator, and in professional and policy development in the Australian vocational education system, and now works as an academic at Griffith University, Australia. He investigates learning through and for work, the nature of work and working knowledge, and how this knowledge is best learnt. He publishes in journals, sole-authored books (*Learning Through Work*: *Strategies for Effective Practice*; *Work, Change and Workers*) and edited volumes (*Work, Subjectivity and Learning; Emerging Perspectives of Work and Learning*), and is the editor-in-chief of *Vocations and Learning*.

Sally Brooks (Royal Melbourne Institute of Technology, Australia) Sally Brooks is the manager of the Career Development and Employment Service at RMIT University. She has over 20 years' experience as a careers counsellor/educator. Currently, Sally is developing a Career Development Learning (CDL) Framework for RMIT and her service has a strong focus on eLearning/online resources for WIL academic staff wishing to integrate CDL into their programmes. Sally has had a 10-year involvement in the teaching, development and course coordination of 'Careers that Work.' From 2000 to 2002 Sally worked as a lecturer in the Faculty of Business Professional Skills Program – a programme that places students in industry projects and develops their management, leadership, teamwork and professional skills. From 2005 to 2009 Sally was the Victorian/Tasmanian State President of National Association of Graduate Careers Advisory Services, and a member of its national management committee.

Jennifer Cartmel (Griffith University, Australia) Dr Jennifer Cartmel is an academic in the School of Human Services and Social Work, Griffith University, Australia whose teaching responsibilities focus on child and family studies and include courses with embedded field education undertaken in a variety of children's services and human services organisations. She is the recipient of an Australian award for university teaching *For reconceptualising practicum experiences for students of early childhood education to facilitate critical reflection of their own practice and that of others*. As well as teaching practitioners she has worked in a range of children's services, preschools and primary schools including a hospital school. She has a particular interest in the many facets of school-aged care settings in Australian and overseas.

Natalie Gamble (Queensland University of Technology, Australia) Natalie Gamble is a project manager and researcher based in the Faculty of Law and the Faculty of Education at Queensland University of Technology, Australia. She has qualifications in organisational psychology and is interested in the preparedness of graduates for professional practice in a range of disciplines. Natalie has a background in the coordination and administration of work-integrated learning (WIL) programmes and is interested in WIL, generic skills, curriculum design and reflective practice. She is currently working on two Australian Learning and Teaching Council-funded projects – the first exploring the development of a capstone experience for undergraduate law students, and the second considering the development of a curriculum-wide approach to reflective writing and reflective practice in undergraduate tertiary degrees.

Pauline Glover (Flinders University, Australia) Associate Professor Pauline Glover has more than 41 years' experience as a midwife in the Australian healthcare system. She has worked as a clinician, educator and researcher in the healthcare system and now works as an academic at Flinders University Australia where she is course coordinator for midwifery programmes. She investigates student learning and the application of theory to practice in the workplace. She is a past editor of the professional journal of the Australian College of Midwives. She is a current reviewer for *Women and Birth*, *Contemporary Nurse* and *Health Sociology Review*.

Amanda Henderson (Queensland Health and Griffith University, Australia) Amanda Henderson is Nursing Director (Education) at Princess Alexandra Hospital, Queensland, Australia, and supervises education initiatives and directives across Metro South Queensland Health (over 5,000 nursing staff). She also holds title of Professor, Griffith Health, Griffith University, Australia, and is an Associate Fellow of the Australian Learning and Teaching Council. Amanda has a strong clinical, education and research background, having worked across both clinical and academic settings. Her scholarship is focused on the establishment of clinical settings that promote the development and utilisation of healthcare knowledge that can ultimately impact on patient care. She has an outstanding international publication record in leading nursing and health journals.

Brian Jolly (Monash University, Australia) A graduate in psychology, Brian Jolly began working in medical education in 1972. In 1981 he completed a Master's degree in medical education, and in 1994 a PhD for work on clinical education at Maastricht University, the Netherlands. He has over 130 peer-reviewed publications, has edited two books and contributed chapters to many more. His Hirsch 'h-index' is currently 18. He is deputy editor of the journal *Medical Education*. In January 2002 he became Professor of Medical Education and Director, Centre for Medical and Health Sciences Education, Monash University. He was on the Federal Ministerial Steering Committee for the recently published Australian Medical Education Study, and in 2009 co-hosted the Ottawa Conference on Medical Education – Ozzawa 2008.

Jenny Keating (Monash University, Australia) Professor Jenny Keating is a physiotherapist and inaugural head of the Department of Physiotherapy at Monash University. She is the course convenor of the Bachelor of Physiotherapy (BPT) and BPT (Honours) and has led the team who developed and continue to refine these new and innovative programmes. In addition to her research activity, Prof. Keating teaches research methods and statistical analysis (around 100 h per year) to BPT students and supervises HDR and honours students. She encourages and supports department staff to evaluate the effects of curriculum changes, particularly those that advance the skills that graduates require to deliver effective health services.

Anna Lichtenberg (University of Wollongong, Australia) Dr Anna Lichtenberg is currently with Deakin University. She has worked at Edith Cowan University for 20 years, in teacher education and as coordinator of career education programmes. Anna is a member of editorial board of the *Australian Journal of Career Development* and has supported professional development of career practitioners through active involvement in professional association activities, career conferences and workshops. She has conducted research and management in a number of career development projects and, since retiring from ECU, has continued working in teacher education and career development at the University of Notre Dame and Victoria University, as well as having ongoing involvement in Australian Careers Service projects.

Sue McAllister (Flinders University, Australia) Dr Sue McAllister has more than 25 years' experience as a speech pathologist, clinical educator, project manager and academic. Her research interests include investigating the nature of professional competency and strategies to support its development through effective university and workplace-based learning, teaching and assessment strategies.

Peter McIlveen (University of Southern Queensland, Australia) Dr Peter McIlveen is with the Faculty of Education at the University of Southern Queensland, Australia. He teaches career development studies and adult learning and coordinates that university's graduate degree in higher education practice. His research interests include the design and evaluation of career development practices (e.g. career counselling, career education) and the development of theoretical frameworks of career and work identity. He is a representative on the Career Industry Council of Australia, editor of the *Australian Journal of Career Development*, and a founding member of Career Development Research Australia. He has held national leadership positions, including vice-president of the Career Industry Council of Australia and President of the National Association of Graduate Careers Advisory Services.

Elizabeth Molloy (Monash University, Australia) Dr Elizabeth Molloy is a senior lecturer at the School of Primary Health Care and the Department of Physiotherapy at Monash University. Dr Molloy coordinates the Unit for Educational Research in the Health Professions in the Masters Degree and teaches into the Graduate Certificate in Health Professional Education. She provides curricular consultation within the Faculty of Medicine, Nursing and Health Sciences at Monash University and has published research on feedback, professional transitions and the role of practitioners and university-based educators in facilitating active student learning. She has recently published a book with Elsevier entitled *Clinical Education in the Health Professions* targeting a multiprofessional audience. She works as a physiotherapist in clinical practice and is team physiotherapist for the Australian Athletics Team.

Jennifer Newton (Monash University, Australia) Dr Jennifer Newton is registered nurse and midwife with an extensive background in clinical and nursing education gained in Australia and England. She now works as a senior research fellow at Monash University and has spent the last decade investigating knowledge development in nursing, graduate transitions, reflective practice and workplace learning. She has numerous journal publications and international conference presentations and is on the editorial board of *Reflective Practice* journal.

Cherene Ockerby (Southern Health, Melbourne, Australia) Cherene Ockerby holds an Honours Degree in Psychology. She has extensive experience as a research assistant working at Southern Health, Melbourne since 2003 and is currently positioned in the Deakin – Southern Health Nursing Research Centre. Her work ranges from undertaking literature reviews and questionnaire design through to data collection, data analysis and report writing, and contributing to publications and conference presentations. Cherene was a member of an ARC Linkage project team that investigated workplace learning in nursing.

Maree O'Keefe (University of Adelaide, Australia) Associate Professor Maree O'Keefe is an educator, researcher and practising paediatrician. She is the Associate Dean Learning and Teaching in the Faculty of Health Sciences at the University of Adelaide, and an Australian Learning and Teaching Council Discipline Scholar. Her research interests include consumer participation in medical education, interprofessional education, student learning in clinical environments and learning outcomes in health.

Deborah Peach (Queensland University of Technology, Australia) Dr Deborah Peach is Director Work-Integrated Learning (WIL), Faculty of Built Environment and Engineering at QUT. Over many years Deborah has made practical and theoretical contributions in the fields of academic staff development, real world learning (RWL), WIL, graduate attributes, generic skills, and pre-service teacher education. She is co-author of The WIL Report: A Scoping Study (2009); recipient of a 2009 ALTC Citation for learning and teaching; and a Fellow of the University of Surrey Centre for Professional Training and Education (SCEPTrE). Deborah is an executive member of the Australian Collaborative Education Network (ACEN) and is the Chair of the ACEN Queensland State Chapter.

Martin Smith (University of Wollongong, Australia) Martin Smith has worked in secondary and higher education roles at the interface between education and the world of work for 25 years. Currently employed as Head, Careers Central at the University of Wollongong, he has held national leadership roles within professional bodies such as the National Association of Graduate Careers Advisory Services (Past President) and Graduate Careers Australia (Director). Examining the contribution of career development learning to work-integrated learning has been a recent research focus. He was awarded a Citation from the Australian Learning and Teaching Council in 2007 and led a national programme which received a Business Higher Education Round Table award for collaboration in 2003.

Ieva Stupans (University of New England, Australia) Professor Ieva Stupans has worked as a pharmacy academic for over 20 years. Her special interests are curriculum design and experiential learning.

Linda Sweet (Flinders University, Australia) Dr Linda Sweet has more than 20 years' experience as a nurse and midwife in the Australian healthcare context. She has worked as a clinician, manager, an academic educator in nursing and midwifery, a clinical educator for undergraduate students, and more recently in health professional educator development. In addition to her educational interests, she has a strong interest in women's health. Dr Sweet investigates clinical learning for health professional students across many different practice models. She is also a sub-editor of the journal *Women and Birth*, and on the editorial board of the *Global Journal of Health Science*. She is a member of, and on the clinical advisory group for, the Australian College of Midwives.

Peter Torjul (Flinders University, Australia) Peter Torjul is a Section Head with responsibility for the Careers and Employer Liaison Centre (Careers, Internship, Graduate Skill Development and Employer Liaison) and Admissions/Student Recruitment (including widening participation) at Flinders University. He has an interest in the application of career development and career management across the student experience, from pre-recruitment through to post-graduation. Peter is a member of the Flinders University College of Distinguished Educators and was previously vice-president of the National Association of Graduate Careers Advisory Services.

Joanne Tyler (Monash University, Australia) Joanne Tyler is Director Employment and Career Development at Monash University, Australia. She has held a number of senior roles including periods as a Director of Graduate Careers Australia; President of the National Association of Graduate careers Advisory Services; founding and executive member of the Career Industry Council of Australia; management committee member of Australian Association of Graduate Employers; and founding and previously executive member of Australian Collaborative Education Network. Joanne worked on development of the Victoria University commitment to embed learning drawn from workplace and community settings in all courses. She has also been responsible for oversight of the post-graduate careers education courses at RMIT. Joanne was awarded a 2007 Carrick Citation (now Australian Learning and Teaching Council) for her work in embedding employability into the curriculum through industry linkages. Her current focus is on building career development learning into the curriculum at Monash University.

Chapter 1
Promoting Professional Learning: Integrating Experiences in University and Practice Settings

Stephen Billett and Amanda Henderson

1.1 New Educational Challenges for Professional Learning

Currently, there is a growing interest in considering how best to assist the learning for professional occupations across universities worldwide. This interest is arising from the increased emphasis within higher education institutions on programmes that aim to prepare students for specific occupational outcomes usually for the professions, and growing expectations that these graduates will be job ready and able to engage in and move smoothly into effectively practising their profession (e.g. Department of Innovation Universities and Skills, 2008; Universities Australia, 2008). Consequently, today, university graduates are increasingly expected to possess the capacities to make a smooth transition into effective professional practice. All of this requires educational programmes that can develop occupationally specific forms of conceptual, procedural, and dispositional capacities that comprise the canonical knowledge of the occupation, something of an understanding about the particular manifestation of that knowledge needed to meet the situational requirements of the circumstances in which they will practise, as well as a set of capacities associated with being self-directed in their learning, working both independently and interdependently, and adopting a reflexively critical capacity that will permit them to monitor, evaluate, and improve practice across working life.

Not surprisingly, therefore, higher education institutions are now increasingly expected to organise curriculum and utilise pedagogies that can realise these three kinds of expectations. These expectations come from government, industry, professional bodies, and, increasingly, students themselves who invest time and money in their degree programmes. Given this focus upon the occupational practice and the need to provide experiences that can assist the development of the conceptual, procedural, and dispositional attributes required to effectively enact occupational practice, it is understandable that there has been a growing interest in providing students with learning experiences within the settings where these occupations are practised,

S. Billett (✉)
School of Education and Professional Studies, Griffith University, Brisbane,
QLD 4112, Australia
e-mail: s.billett@griffith.edu.au

S. Billett, A. Henderson (eds.), *Developing Learning Professionals*, Professional and Practice-based Learning 7, DOI 10.1007/978-90-481-3937-8_1,

as well as those within university settings. Indeed, experiences in practice settings are increasingly seen as being indispensable components of the higher educational curriculum for many sectors. The realisation that participation in university-based activities and interactions alone is insufficient to develop the competence required for effective professional practice is far from new and has long since led to the inclusion of practice-based experiences in courses of professional preparation (Jolly & Macdonald, 1989). Yet, experiences in practice settings may still be seen as largely providing opportunities for students to merely practise what they have learnt in the academy, or to develop the skills for practice, rather than these settings being accepted as providing rich and legitimate learning experiences in their own right (Billett, 2001; Boud & Solomon, 2001), and, as such, making particular and salient contributions to the development of professional competence (Henderson, Twentyman, Heel, & Lloyd, 2006). Moreover, despite the growing recognition of the learning potential arising from them, it is perhaps the exception to identify circumstances where students' experiences in practice-based settings are seen as being a legitimate and integral component of the students' higher education curriculum (Billett, 2009). However, attempts to maximise the knowledge learnt from practice settings through their integration with what is taught and learnt through experiences within the university have yet to become a central curriculum or pedagogical tenet of higher education. The contributions provided in this volume seek to contribute to redressing this situation through their considerations of how higher education student learning can be generated in ways that support the integration of experiences in both settings.

Here, understandings are advanced about practices associated with how the integration of student's experiences across the university and practice settings might best proceed in assisting realise educational purposes associated with preparing graduates who are adept and agentic professional practitioners. These goals are realised through drawing on the findings of a series of projects conducted in Australia that have investigated diverse aspects of work-integrated arrangements and commonly have sought to develop robust professional practitioners. In considering these projects, this volume provides a platform to understand and appraise diverse perspectives and practices that seek to integrate students' experiences within higher educational institutions with those that are encountered within practice settings across a range of discipline areas, yet within the same national higher education context.

So, the collective aims of this volume are focused on identifying, discussing, and elaborating processes through which professional learning can be effectively promoted through the intentional and guided integration of learning experiences across university and practice settings. As noted, this is increasingly an important consideration for higher education in advanced and emerging economies. Across a range of countries, programmes in universities are being positioned as 'higher vocational education', with expectations that graduates will enjoy smooth transitions to professional practice (Department of Innovation Universities and Skills, 2008). Indeed, the progressive shift in the emphasis in university programmes in many countries away from liberal arts (Lomas, 1997) and more towards preparation for specific occupations has led pejoratively to descriptions of universities as now primarily being involved in 'higher vocational education'. As noted, aligned with this positioning is an increased interest in and emphasis on work-integrated learning within higher education, albeit taking different forms across different countries and universities within countries. Some will see this educational focus as a slight, others a description of a changing focus for higher education meeting particular social and economic goals. Yet, regardless of the way this discussion runs, a focused consideration of the purposes, procedures, and aspirations of higher education and to what degree these are supported or imperilled by these changes is now urgently warranted. Certainly, meeting the high expectations of governments, employers, and students represents a significant educational challenge to those who work in higher education and seek to organise and enact effective experiences for their students. There are important questions to be addressed not only about the educational worth of these experiences but also about how best should the integration of these experiences occur within higher education to approximate or realise the expectations of those who sponsor and employ graduates and make judgements about provisions of higher education. Arguably, these kinds of outcomes are what most higher education students want, employers increasingly demand, and governments expect. Yet, to get close to realising these kinds of outcomes within higher education programmes requires the selection and organisation of learning experiences that can best develop these occupational capacities. All of these imperatives are leading to a growing interest in and an emphasis on work-integrated learning within higher education, albeit taking different forms across different disciplines, institutions, and countries.

Certainly, the educational challenges arising from these demands are for universities to prepare their graduates for specific occupations and for these graduates to enjoy successful and smooth transitions to instances of professional practice, which cannot be known until the graduate is employed within them. Yet, fulfilling this expectation constitutes a very difficult educational goal; because the particular requirements for professional practice can differ quite widely across occupations, as do the settings in which practitioners work. The work undertaken by nurses in a major teaching hospital within a metropolitan capital may be quite different from that undertaken by their counterparts in a small rural hospital, health-care centre in a remote community, or in a doctor's surgery as a practice nurse. Moreover, in contrast to the specific requirements of the settings in which these individuals will work, there are now growing demands for graduates to meet the requirements of national standards associated with professional practice. The educational provisions for some occupations have long been highly ordered and include regulated arrangements for practice experiences (e.g. teaching, nursing). Other occupations follow different kinds of long-standing, practice-based arrangements (e.g. medicine, physiotherapy, accountancy, law). However, far more, and perhaps the majority of, disciplines have practice-based arrangements that are enacted on less structured and organised bases than supervised placements in preparatory occupation programmes for a range of disciplines. So, there is a need to develop the canonical knowledge of each profession (i.e. the knowledge required by all who practise that occupation), and also a requirement for this knowledge to be learnt in ways that make it adaptable to the practices that graduates will encounter during their courses and directly upon graduation in particular practice settings (Billett, 2009). Fortunately, these kinds of purposes and processes are not wholly novel to higher education. Moreover, they have long been exercised by the North American co-op movement, through its provision of extensive periods of workplace placements (e.g. internships) and also through practicums in such courses as medicine, teaching, nursing, and physiotherapy across diverse settings for a long time (e.g. Boud & Solomon, 2001).

It is for these reasons that there is a need for graduates to have practice-based experiences throughout their programmes of study. But, more than having access to experiences in practice settings, importantly, these formative and constructive experiences should be effectively integrated within the curriculum so that the contributions from both settings can assist in developing both the canonical occupational knowledge and the understanding of how this knowledge might be applied differently across a range of professional settings. Indeed, more than simply being settings in which to experience the occupational practice and apply what has been learnt in university settings, practice settings provide essential learning experiences in their own right (Billett, 2001). Consequently, practice-based experiences need to be positioned to strengthen and augment what is learnt through experiences in educational institutions, as well as make their own contributions. Yet, effective participation in and learning from experiences in university and practice settings requires a certain set of personal capacities, including the capacity to be an agentic learner. This capacity is also central to what constitutes an effective professional practitioner: that is someone with the capacity to be able to independently appraise the processes and outcomes of their practice, and make judgements about its efficacy and how it might be improved.

Of course, and understandably, some educators view these changes as being problematic and being the antithesis of what should constitute higher education. There are also concerns that the imperatives of particular interests (e.g. workplaces) will be privileged over other educational purposes, specifically those often associated with university courses. These purposes include developing broadly adaptable knowledge and critical stances, rather than meeting particular sets of social and economic goals. These are important reservations and need to be taken seriously, not the least because they are central to both what differentiates higher education but also because these critical faculties are those required by professionals to reflect on, monitor, and enhance their practice in relatively self-regulated ways across their working lives. Indeed, these different purposes are not necessarily as inconsistent or irreconcilable as they might first seem to those concerned with a focus on liberal education. Paid work, and particularly that practised by the professions, requires the capacity for the constant adaptation of knowledge and criticality in practice because its requirements are distinct and subject to constant change (Billett, 2006). Moreover, the capacities for professional work go beyond technical knowledge or ways of knowing (e.g. Aristotle's concept of techne or applied knowledge (Stevenson, 1994)) and are associated with the exercise of critical facilities within domains of occupational practice. Hence, it is important for there to be a focus on developing criticality as part of these higher education provisions. It follows, therefore, that there are important and urgent issues associated with understanding, identifying, and utilising the educational worth of authentic experiences and proposing how the integration of these experiences might best proceed within university courses.

In all, we need to be informed when addressing the question: How should we proceed as higher educators? Offered here are a range of perspectives drawn from a series of Australian projects that have investigated processes through which the integrations of experiences in educational and practice settings might proceed to realise these kinds of goals. The contributions are drawn from projects that sought to identify the scope and bases for advancing work-integrated learning across the higher education system nationally and those that investigated curriculum and pedagogic practices to support that integration. Collectively, what is advanced in these contributions comprises the findings and synthesis of a series of projects that are seeking to inform the understanding about the significance of integrating experiences in practice and academic settings. Given the interest, internationally, within higher education to utilise and effectively integrate into higher education curriculum experiences from practice settings, the contributions here should attract a wide readership. Its strengths will be found in its conceptual premises, elaborations and synthesis, and the use of actual incidents of practice to elaborate these premises and advance curriculum and pedagogic practices from a range of areas of professional practice.

1.1.1 Projects Informing This Volume

The contributions of this book focus on the kinds of experiences that can best assist the effective initial preparation of professional practitioners, including a smooth transition into practice and the development of 'learning professionals'. This is achieved through the consideration of conceptual premises for the initial learning of professional knowledge and the kinds of contributions to that learning which can be provided through experiences in both educational institutions and through authentic practice-based experiences. These considerations are informed by a series of studies of professional learning. First is a 3-year project on improving the learning practices within hospital settings for trainee nurses and by preceptor nurses (Chapter 3). Second is a multipart project that investigated instances of integrating experiences across university and practice settings in order to address specific learning-related issues in the professional fields of midwifery, physiotherapy, nursing, and human services (Chapters 4, 5, 6, and 7). A separate but related study explored the integration of joint practicum experiences of medical and nursing students, and further extended students' authentic practice (Chapter 8), and one focused on the relations between health-care organisations and medical students' experiences (Chapter 11). Each of these studies exercised particular kinds of curriculum and pedagogic responses to address discipline-specific teaching and learning problems and, thereby, provided useful and specific findings that can inform the provision of teaching and learning experiences within higher education. Two further studies are incorporated here. The first comprised a study of how the student service function in universities might best assist students' engagement in work-related learning experiences (Chapter 9). The sixth study comprised a national project that sought to understand the scope, purposes, characteristics, and effectiveness of work-integrated learning experiences across a range of Australian universities (Chapter 10). Together, these studies provide largely qualitative-based accounts to understand the learning potential of integrating experiences in both academic and practice settings. Collectively, these studies provide a current, focused, and helpful base to understand the prospects for enhancing professional learning through the integration of these experiences. The support provided by the Australian Research Council and the Australian Learning and Teaching Council in funding these projects deserves to be acknowledged here.

1.1.2 Conceptual Premises for Appraising the Worth of Integrating Experiences

The contributions that flow from these studies are advanced within each chapter and captured in summary here. However, given the ambitious educational challenge confronting university educators in preparing graduates for smooth transitions to professional practice, it is important to provide a platform from which considerations, deliberations, and practice might best progress. This platform needs to include a consideration of the kinds of educational goals to be realised and the premises for considering how the contributions from experiences in academic and practice settings can be utilised and integrated, and then needs to identify the premises for their integration. Accordingly, the next chapter – *Integrating Experiences in Workplace and University Settings: A Conceptual Perspective* – offers some bases by which this appraisal might progress. It does this by first proposing the kinds and forms of knowledge required to be developed for performance in professional practice. These kinds of knowledge have been identified through extensive enquiries within different fields of psychology and comprise the domain-specific conceptual, procedural, and dispositional knowledge of the particular occupational field. Conceptual knowledge comprises facts, concepts, and propositions which are all statable. This knowledge, which is also often referred to as propositional or declarative knowledge, ranges from simple factual knowledge to richly interlinked sets of facts and propositions. Indeed, depth of conceptual knowledge is held to be about associations rather than merely the possession of massive amounts of knowledge. Importantly, these links and associations between concepts and propositions perhaps most likely arise through episodes of experience which bring separate and sometimes disparate ideas together through their application in practice. Procedural knowledge comprises the knowledge through which we do things, including thinking or acting. It is far less easy to state than is with conceptual knowledge. Indeed, it is likely that when we attempt to state procedures, we are likely giving accounts of something that we believe is occurring, yet to which we may not have complete access. Again, there are different kinds and perhaps a hierarchy within procedures. There are simple specific procedures that comprise specific tasks or task execution, and then there are strategic procedures which comprise processes through which options are considered and evaluated, and courses of action progressed. Often, the development of procedural capacities arises through individuals learning specific procedures and then progressing to use their procedures in more strategic ways. Following these forms of knowledge there are the dispositions, such as interest, values, and intentionality, that direct individuals' efforts in particular ways. These dispositions are important because they shape how individuals conceptualise things and the degree by which they direct effort when they enact tasks. Hence, these are the premises upon which individuals direct their conscious thinking and acting (Perkins, Jay, & Tishman, 1993). Important for considering effective occupational practices is that beyond these kinds of knowledge, there at least two domain-specific forms of that knowledge that have quite distinct characteristics.

These forms comprise the canonical knowledge of the occupation and, importantly, situated instances of how this knowledge is manifested in particular settings. That is, there is a domain associated with the knowledge that is required for an occupation: the canonical knowledge of that occupation. This is the kind of knowledge which all practitioners are expected to possess and utilise. Then, there is the domain of knowledge that comprises the requirements to be effective in particular situations; that is an understanding of the goals for, requirements of, likely processes to be effective in, and means of engaging in a particular instance of occupational practice. In many ways, the canonical domain of knowledge is abstract and dis-embedded from particular instances of practice. It stands as a set of propositions, dispositions, and procedures that exist as an ideal and a requirement. Yet, it is only when these propositions, dispositions, and procedures are enacted or aligned with a particular instance of practice do the requirements for performance become real (Billett, 2001). So, whereas the worth of an individual's knowledge in a university setting might be assessed against canonical requirements, such as those stated in curriculum documents or professional standards, it is the capacity to perform against situational requirements in a particular practice setting that will be the basis upon which a graduate is assessed. Therefore, a key consideration for developing occupational competence is how contributions of experiences in academic and practice settings are appraised in terms of how they separately, and also when integrated, might best secure the kinds and forms of knowledge to be learnt. In this way, considerations of curriculum need to include how to identify the best fit between the experiences provided and the required knowledge. This consideration goes beyond what is afforded by the two settings and the integration of their contributions to include learners' necessary contributions to the learning of these forms and kinds of knowledge. A key consideration for both curriculum and pedagogy arising here is that an emphasis on the learner needs to be accentuated, perhaps more than it is when they are positioned as being a student within a higher education course. Students as learners should always be centre stage. However, currently, this is not always the case, particularly when concerns about teaching predominate and easy assumptions about the relationship between teaching and learning are prosecuted. In particular, in these kinds of curriculum arrangements – with students engaging in experiences in both the educational and practice settings – it is these students who will have to construe and construct their knowledge, usually in circumstances without access to teachers. Therefore, discussions about curriculum and pedagogy need to extend beyond considerations of what is enacted as experiences for students, and include their epistemological development as agentic learners. Therefore, it will not be sufficient to consider the development of appropriate curriculum and pedagogies. Rather, it will be necessary also to consider the development of agentic personal epistemologies.

To conceptualise the process of integration, it is proposed that three specific conceptions may be helpful. First, the integrations are seen as being derived from experiences in two distinct kinds of social settings (i.e. the educational institution and the practice setting). It is often assumed that distinct forms of knowledge are learnt in each of the settings (i.e. theory in one and practice in the other). However, it is likely that the development of conceptual, procedural, and dispositional knowledge and in both their canonical and situational forms can arise from experiences in both kinds of settings, typically when brought together. However, there can be no certainty about this because what is provided in educational institutions would be quite distinct, as is the case with experiences in practice settings. In this situational account, it is presumed that the experiences of both will contribute towards the smooth transition to practice. The second view – the personal constructivist perspective – is that the focus should be on how the individual makes sense of what they experience across both settings and that ultimately it is the individual experience that is central to how individuals reconcile and integrate what they encounter in both settings. This perspective is consonant with a phenomenological view of learning. Here, the construction of the personal experience is seen to be the centre of considerations of curriculum and pedagogy, and this view leads to consideration of the importance of personal epistemologies. However, because it is important that considerations be given to the social settings in which individuals engage and learn from practices that have historical geneses, and also the importance of the personal epistemologies which shaped how they learn, it is necessary for a conception which encompasses both sets of contributions. Consequently, the third perspective – a socio-personal account of integration – comprises an amalgam of these different perspectives. That is, it acknowledges the contributions of both the social and personal world and the ways in which social and personal agencies play key roles in accessing and learning, and then refining and developing further the knowledge required for professional practice. This then leads into a consideration of how curriculum and pedagogy practices might best be organised to support this learning.

1.2 Integrating Practice and University Experiences: Curriculum and Pedagogy Practices

Having considered these conceptual premises for students integrating experiences across practice and university settings, it is helpful to understand curriculum and pedagogic practices which might support such integrations. Of course, there are a variety of ways in which curriculum and pedagogy are defined and used. Consequently, it is useful to say something about use of these terms here before advancing accounts of their utility in integrating these experiences. Curriculum here is taken as the overall ordering of students' experiences. This includes a consideration of the kinds of experiences and also their sequencing and alignment with the educational goals. For instance, the typical practice in many higher education programmes is for students to engage in practicum experiences towards the end of the programmes. In this way, the curriculum proposes that specific forms of knowledge are best learnt in the university setting and that these need to come before students engage in practice-based experiences. Yet, there might be reasons for providing those experiences far earlier, for instance, to permit students to understand something of the occupational practice that they have selected, or for them to engage in tasks that assist them understand the roles that they may ultimately take (e.g. student teaches acting as teacher aides and nurses acting as hospital orderlies). Pedagogy here is taken as the means for enabling and enriching those experiences, usually through the intervention of another or more experienced partner (e.g. teacher and workplace expert). Hence, the kind of activities which university educators provide to assist students understand the purposes and outcomes of the practicum experiences can be seen as being pedagogic. At one level, these can include the use of interventions before, during, and after the student's engagement in practice-based experiences (Billett, 2009). At another level, these activities refer to the kinds of specific interventions that educators and others might utilise. For instance, the use of focus groups, learning circles, critical dialogues, etc., both within university and practice settings, all stand as examples of these kinds of interventions. Yet, pedagogic practices are not restricted to experiences within educational settings, as many such interventions are also enacted in workplaces. Much of the guidance provided by more experienced workers is of this kind. So, in these ways, pedagogy is seen as enriching the experiences provided by activities in both practice and educational settings. Also, not surprisingly, there is sometimes an overlap between experiences that are ordered as curriculum and enriched by pedagogy. For instance, at the commencement and end of each shift, nurses usually engage in what is referred to as the 'handover' process. This is a routine practice where the patients are discussed and their condition, its treatment, and the patient responses to the treatment are considered and appraised. This process represents a rich opportunity for learning about nursing and health care in general. This is because the nurses, and then the nurse students participating, engage their knowledge in considering the patient's case and through this consideration and discussions are able to exercise and appraise their knowledge, consider the perspectives of others, and develop further understandings. This experience is in part curriculum, because it is an experience provided through engaging in nursing work. That is, although it is not specifically intended as a learning event, it needs to serve this purpose for the continuity of patient care, yet also promotes the learning of those who are participating within these meetings. Yet, it is also pedagogic because it is an intervention that serves to enrich the learning experience, in particular, through the opportunity to engage with others, reflect on existing knowledge, and also appraise individuals' knowledge against what others are proposing.

The contributions of this book do much to elaborate the understanding of how such experiences arise both in curriculum terms and through pedagogic practices. Moreover, much of the considerations within some of the chapters are associated with how the sets of experiences in both education and practice settings might best be drawn together, reconciled, and advanced. For instance, in the chapter led by Jennifer Newton – *Preparing Nurses and Engaging Preceptors* –it is advanced that the experiences in practice settings are essential in the preparation of student nurses to become effective functioning nursing practitioners. It focuses on the potential of preceptors (i.e. experienced nurses who assist student or junior nurses) to enable and enrich the clinical experience of student nurses. This proposition is well acknowledged within nursing practice and also with the literature. A 3-year study examining workplace learning in nursing, in particular the preceptorship model, accentuated differences in novices and experienced practitioners' professional learning experiences. The affordances offered to student nurses by the clinical learning environment, and their capacity to engage with this environment, were critical to the quality of their learning experience. The findings highlight the intricacies of workplace learning in relation to individuals' dispositions, the level of engagement with available learning opportunities, and the receptiveness of the workplace to the novice nurse. Factors associated with creating learning opportunities, outcomes of the novice's increasing independence and socialisation as a team member, and the negotiation of intergenerational differences that compound the complexities of a health-care profession are accentuated in the quality of the support and guidance afforded and how individuals engage with those affordances. Much of the support was provided as part of everyday work activity by preceptors, and also by other and more experienced nurses, as they worked together on the shifts. The support assisted the students to effectively participate in the ward's activities, engage in nursing, and also learn through these experiences. Then, this support was also useful in extending the students' knowledge about and capacities to practise nursing. So, in these ways, whether from an official preceptor or an experienced nurse, the students' professional learning and important integration of what they had learned in the university was both enabled and extended by these co-workers. Yet, in addition, the students provided evidence of how their ability to engage with these workers was also premised on how they themselves elected to engage in the workplace and with these sources of support and guidance. This exercise of agency extends to how these individuals decide to engage with others and reflect upon what they have learnt within the university and clinical settings. What emerges from the study is the importance of both preceptors, for whom supporting junior nurses is part of their role, and experienced nurses, who appeared to be exercising a professional obligation by supporting student or junior nurses with whom they work, in supporting these nurses' learning. Yet, what was evident in situations when neither preceptors nor experts were available or supportive is that this support can never be wholly relied upon, because it may not afford students in particular settings. Moreover, it is unlikely that the agency of students will be sufficient to bridge the gap, because much of what they need to know requires access to more experienced partners. Hence, beyond the curriculum and pedagogic practices demonstrated here are the needs for interventions in education institutions to support the development of this agency. As has been noted (Billett, 2009), a consideration of pedagogic interventions before, during, and after the practicum periods is likely to be helpful in enabling and enriching students' experiences in practice settings, and can extend and assist the integration of experiences in both of those settings.

In their chapter, entitled *Targeted Preparation for Clinical Practice*, Liz Molloy and Jenny Keating refer to a particular set of experiences designed to prepare physiotherapy students for long periods of practicum experiences. These authors developed and enacted a 1-week transition programme that aimed to enhance students' preparation for the demands of clinical experience and learning. The aims of the transition programme included (i) making transparent the expectations of students taking clinical education and (ii) advancing student knowledge and skills in applied adult learning to facilitate negotiating the complex challenges and uncertainty of the clinical environment and physiotherapy work. Yet, again the dual considerations of both what the programme afforded and how students engaged with it emerged as a key issue. Students reported high levels of satisfaction with the transition programme. However, focus groups revealed a disjunction between the goals of the intended curriculum organised by educators and students' bases for participating in the programme. Educators designed the transition programme to provide learners with agency through the development of generic skills in communication, leadership, and critical thinking. In contrast, students' priorities reflected a 'survival focus', and a preoccupation with the attainment and demonstration of technical skills, the application of which was required for their forthcoming practicum experiences. Survey results supported that students placed greater value on discipline-specific practical classes than activities designed to promote generic skill development such as lectures on adult learning principles and leadership in practice. This finding was reinforced by the preference for activities promoting technical skill development. Students acknowledged the benefit of educators and 4th-year students providing heuristic or 'tricks of the trade' information during the transition week, including information on how to negotiate the supervisory relationship and what to expect from assessment procedures within the week-long programme. Hence, an element of student agency might be to actively ignore what educators intend and intentionally focus on their own priorities. Indeed, as students engage in a range of activities simultaneously to their higher education studies and make judgements about their engagement amongst those activities, it seems that they are becoming increasingly time jealous. That is, they are making judgements and decisions about how to use their time strategically, to meet their needs. Consequently, the sequencing and timing of experiences may need to accommodate the kind of challenges which students are immediately facing, and use these challenges as a key means for organising the curriculum (i.e. the kind and sequence of experiences to be offered to students). In this way, pedagogically, to align student and educator intentions more closely, it may be better to prepare teaching and learning activities that promote skill development in the context of clinical activities where students perceive that they are attaining tangible skills with utility and transferability. Physiotherapy students praised learning activities they perceived as being relevant to their learning and the imminent requirements for them to practise physiotherapy in health-care settings. What was common about these experiences is that they focused on immediate imperatives associated with students' time and goals.

A similar finding, which also shaped students' engagement in intentional pedagogic practices, is reported in Linda Sweet and Pauline Glover's chapter entitled *Optimising the Follow Through Experience for Midwifery Learning.* These authors discuss their engagement with students in the midwifery course and the use of teaching strategies (i.e. reflective logs) to assist these students integrate their experiences within the university with those of their engagement with birthing mothers. Indeed, these students became both time poor and time jealous as a result of progress demands made upon them by the professional body that will accredit them as practising midwives. The Australian College of Midwives standards for the Bachelor of Midwifery mandate that a significant portion of clinical learning be achieved through a follow-through education (FTE) programme. The FTE programme is a continuity model for midwifery students whereby, in partnership with birthing women, they experience pregnancy and childbirth through the requirement to complete 30 follow-throughs across the 3-year programme. These then become a significant component of the midwife curriculum, and they comprise a significant and, often, compelling set of experiences for the students. The educational intent of these experiences is threefold: (i) engaging students with midwifery work and practices and opportunities to reflect upon them; (ii) developing the capacities to be an effective midwife; and (iii) understanding the nuances and differences within the birthing process. In these ways, there is a deliberate attempt to develop both the canonical knowledge of midwifery and instances of its situated requirements. Nevertheless, as can be imagined, to follow 30 women through the processes leading up to the birth of their children, and to be available to support these women across this period of time and at the birth, is an extremely time-consuming and effortful activity that is achieved through the exclusion of other activities. The midwife educators have the students use reflective logs to enrich their experience of these follow-through experiences. However, given the demands of their study life, including engaging with birthing women, the engagement by students in their reflective logs became increasingly cursory across their follow-through experiences. Therefore, there is a greater requirement to make these experiences worthwhile for the students and as rich and productive as possible. The authors identify a set of pedagogic interventions that may occur before the students engage in their follow-through experiences, during those experiences, and after these experiences. Prior to the students engaging in these activities, it is proposed to provide an orientation to these experiences, and ensure students are equipped with appropriate procedural and conceptual knowledge associated with foundational midwifery practices and an understanding of the different kinds of trajectories along which birthing mothers will progress. During these experiences, the students should engage fully as a member of health-care teams within the scope of their expanding competence, and also be prepared to indicate that there are limits to their competence should they be pressed to engage in activities that exceed these limits. After these experiences, it is proposed to provide students with the opportunity not only to share their experiences with other students to enrich all students' experiences but also for clinical supervision purposes, that is to engage students in critical reflection upon practice that is directed not only towards developing occupational competence but also at taking care of the self.

This issue of taking care of the self is central to the case made by Jennifer Cartmel in her chapter entitled *Preparing Human Services Practitioners*. Students undertaking field placements in human service organisations often encounter routine aspects of human service work that are confronting for novices. Consequently, students may need support in their professional preparation, including ways of addressing and accommodating confronting experiences, so they are prepared for and can respond appropriately to such encounters. In feedback, students often referred to being ill-prepared for the challenges they experienced in their field placements. Hence, enacting a curriculum and teaching practice that support students' engagement with the practicum experience became a key educational goal for this author. Here, university-based teaching strategies that seek to develop personal strategies for effective practice and personal coping are appraised. These strategies are designed to assist students be well-equipped and placed to understand and respond effectively to situations which require them to bring about change for individuals, groups, and communities. Exposing students to real-life scenarios is explored as this teaching approach has the potential to make students resilient as professional practitioners through making them aware of potential confronting situations and the unpredictability of dealing with people who are emotionally or otherwise confronting. However, these strategies may also have the potential to create the opposite outcome. That is, unless carefully managed, they, also, potentially can lead to students being dissuaded from a career in the sector. Consequently, the development of this agentic quality of being able to deal with confronting situations is essential for a productive and healthy professional life in human services. In order to develop these capacities, the author trialled a process of using 'learning circles' as a shared space in which students could come together, supervised by a teacher, before and during their placements. The approach was premised on shared critical reflection. The utility of these activities was supported in the feedback from students in terms of the creation of an environment in which they could share experiences and develop further their understandings, as well as model the important process of clinical supervision which is central to the health and development of workers in this field.

Jennifer Newton also evaluates the use of group sharing and reflection with student nurses in her chapter *Reflective Learning Groups for Student Nurses*. Interacting with other health-care professionals and professionals from other disciplines can be challenging for novice nurses. Recent research reports that new nursing graduates consistently claim to be inadequately prepared for the clinical workplace and the associated responsibilities required as a practising nurse, including interacting with other and more experienced practitioners. The inadequacy of their preparation is held to be the product of a mismatch between experiences provided in the university setting and the requirements for practice in the health-care setting. In particular, the curriculum and pedagogic practices used in university setting are held not to adequately prepare graduates for the transition to their professional role. Thus, new graduates struggle with the tensions between the ide-als they brought into nursing and the reality of professional practice. Some of this misalignment is associated with the distinct activities and interactions occurring in university and health-care settings. Moreover, in particular, the complexity of patient care delivery is increasing as the need to engage with a growing range of professionals in work-intense environments makes processes of engaging and communicating increasingly difficult, particularly for those who are unfamiliar with the terms, norms, and practices being deployed as part of standard everyday work practice. This chapter discusses the facilitation of student nurses' development of their professional role through the process of supported reflection. This is realised through the experiences of six students' participation in a reflective learning group during the final year of their undergraduate degree. Considerations of how the use of reflective learning group supports the development of nursing students as active learners are illustrated through appraisals of the students' engagement in and learn-ing through their participation in such a group. The students, although engaged in workplace environments with many co-workers and other kinds of workers, often reported feeling isolated and overwhelmed by the demands of engaging in such work-intensive environments. However, after they were implemented, the students reported that the reflective learning groups provided the means both before and dur-ing their clinical experiences to share and reflect with peers. The study found that a range of benefits accrued to the students from their participation in these groups. First, their confidence was buttressed by a process of sharing experiences and learn-ing that others were encountering issues similar to those that they experienced. Moreover, these groups provided a safe environment in which students could share their experiences without concerns about how their opinions would be received by experienced practitioners. Second, students reported experiencing transformational learning in the form of perspective shifts arising from discussions with peers, which in many ways augmented the advice that had been provided individually to group members. Students also claimed that the interactions with peers generated capacities to more effectively engage with preceptors and other co-workers, thereby enhanc-ing the basis by which the students could engage in the health-care settings. In all, and along with others, these reflective groups were seen to provide a helpful ped-agogic intervention that supported the student nurses' learning and the formation of a positive identity as a novice nurse. The latter is particularly important to the nursing occupation because there is a high attrition rate arising from poor work-place experiences and a lack of satisfaction with nursing work by newly qualified students.

The studies reported above all focused on the development of professional capac-ities by individual students. Many of the processes proposed to develop these capacities have centred on the use of group activities that feature opportunities for the sharing of experiences and reflections upon individual and collective delib-erations. However, an increasing emphasis in the development of occupational capacities is the specific goal of being able to work within teams. Some go even as far as to suggest that expertise needs to be seen in terms of collective action because, increasingly, individuals' performance is shaped by securing work goals through interacting and working with others.

It is within this context that Amanda Henderson and Heather Alexander discussed the prospects for interprofessional learning within groups of medical and nursing students in clinical environments in their chapter entitled *Engaging and Integrating Medical and Nursing Students in Clinical Learning Environments*. The authors note that limited attention is given to teamwork or building interprofessional relations as part of university courses. Such is the concern for nursing and medicine professionals to work together that efforts to collaborate during their initial professional preparation are being requested by both government and employers. Certainly, within clinical practice settings, effective teamwork is held to be essential for medical and nursing professionals to provide safe and effective patient care. The authors claim that there is evidence that, through team communication and collaboration, health-care effectiveness is improving. Hence, the project reported in this chapter aims to develop communication and collaboration in nursing and medical students and processes of collaborative engagement in clinical settings. However, historically medical and nursing students have been educated and largely practise separately from each other, and in quite distinct ways. Overall, the clinical practice experience for both professional groups is focused on the development of profession-specific knowledge. This is reflected in the structure and supervision during the clinical placements where students are located in the silo of their profession. Further, the authors list a range of institutional barriers for these two kinds of students to come together. Yet, they conclude that there is a common basis for interprofessional communication and working: the patient. Using a strategy of engaging just one medical student with one nursing student in a structured arrangement that focuses on a particular case study and is facilitated by the clinical educator, the authors propose what is claimed as a manageable and sustainable approach to interprofessional learning. The process comprises the two students reading the patient's records and otherwise ascertaining information about their health record. Following this phase, the two students interview patients and discuss with them the reasons for their admission, social circumstances, and programme of care and the availability of support and assistance. After this interview, they engage in a process of discussing their respective roles and obligations towards the patients, before finally discussing the three stages referred to above with a clinical educator. It is proposed that such a set of arrangements are a sustainable response to the various constraints which inhibit medical and nursing students from being brought together on a more regular basis. These curriculum and pedagogic practices are held to be premised on three important sets of factors. First, the availability and enactment of leadership within clinical setting is seen as essential. Second, clinical engagement, which refers to the kinds of opportunities in clinical settings for these arrangements to be enacted and supported by the clinical setting, was enacted. Third, the importance of relevant clinical activities is seen as being central to whether the interprofessional collaborations are successful in educational terms.

1.3 Institutional Practices and Imperatives

The second and shorter set of contributions to this book refers specifically to educational institutions' practices and imperatives to promote professional learning. These contributions refer to the provision of career development preparation and accounts of the ways in which a range of higher education institutions decided to respond to imperatives associated with integrating practice experiences within the higher education curriculum.

In their chapter – *Career Development Learning* – Peter McIlveen, Sally Brooks, Anna Lichtenberg, Martin Smith, Peter Torjul, and Joanne Tyler refer to the role that career development has long played as a set of educational purposes and practices that aim to enhance both personal and societal worth of educational provisions that are closely aligned with paid work. This role has perhaps become increasingly important for all sectors of education as these alignments seem to be commonly sought. Considerations of occupational preparation are increasingly shaping compulsory education in many if not most countries with advanced industrial economies, as the national imperatives for being globally competitive increase, and parents and others seek to position their children most advantageously within well-paid and worthwhile work. Moreover, how occupational preparation proceeds across different countries vocational education is often quite tightly aligned to specific forms of employment, and yet, there are often high levels of non-completion in programmes such as apprenticeships in some countries. This indicates the need for more of the kind of provisions to which McIlveen et al. refer. However, their key focus is on higher education provisions and the development of career self-management by higher education students. In this way, they echo what others have suggested about students needing to be proactive and agentic as both learners and workers. What they argue, and again quite consistently with other views, is the need for students to personalise the direction and purpose of their learning and to be aware of how the different components of the courses might contribute to their career prospects and development. The authors propose that such educational purposes can best be realised through students having workplace experiences and then using these as a platform to identify, consider, and reconcile their goals for their higher education. They propose a process through which this might be realised for students in higher education comprising self-awareness, opportunity awareness, decision making, and transition learning. Self-awareness refers to the students being engaged and reflective in terms of the aims and goals and decision making within higher education programmes. Opportunity awareness refers to the ways in which various opportunities that are afforded to students can serve their purposes, they meet students' needs, and they respond to these opportunities. The appropriateness and focused quality of decision making is the third key quality for students to be self-managed in the development of their careers. Finally, the authors refer to the capacities to effectively negotiate transitions between education and work, different forms of employment, and different employment situations. In this way, they propose a framework for higher education students which seeks to provide them with the kinds of personal capital that will assist them secure the best alignment between their personal interests and capacities, and the world of paid employment in which the majority will spend much of their life.

In their chapter, Deborah Peach and Natalie Gamble report outcomes of a review of practices within 30 higher education institutions in Australia that aimed to engage and utilise work experiences as part of programme provisions to prepare graduates who are job ready. In the aptly named contribution – *Scoping Work-Integrated Learning Purposes, Practices and Outcomes* – they commence by noting that there are a variety of practices and terminologies associated with the current practices within these institutions. Indeed, they note that there is nothing particularly novel about the provision of work experiences for university students, although their specific integration into the curriculum may be innovative for some programmes. Yet, what may be new are the more universal engagements in these kinds of arrangements and also the more specific emphasis on direct employability. Often, programmes that have provided supervised placements have been in a minority and offered in relatively small numbers. However, in an era of mass higher education and growing government and community expectations about graduates being job ready, universities are now considering ways in which they can manage these growing expectations, all within the constraints of existing funding regimes. Not least driving these demands is students wanting relevant and practical experiences. Yet, the scoping study found that the most common reference to work-integrated learning arrangements are those associated with supervised practicums, many of which are premised on cross-institutional agreements (e.g. between faculties of education and schooling departments, and between faculties of nursing and hospitals). But, as noted, these arrangements are available for only a small percentage of higher education students and issues of access are likely to frustrate goals of universal engagement. The authors propose that this new imperative for providing work experiences will likely press all academic areas within universities to build these kinds of partnerships and cross-institutional arrangements. Yet, these are likely to be more or less complex tasks depending upon the kinds of programmes and range of workplaces they serve. For instance, one senior university administrator asked this author 'How are we supposed to find supervised placements for 1500 undergraduate business students?' Hence, outside of situations where there are clearly identifiable partners comes the need to find ways of linking universities with workplaces and managing student's experiences in a way that can accommodate the requirements and resources of mass higher education and also identify different models and approaches which are less resource intensive. Realising all of these matters becomes a key emerging challenge for institutes of higher education because all stakeholders (government, public and private sector, students) and many educators want these kinds of provisions.

Having considered the imperatives of educational institutions, Maree O'Keefe, Sue McAllister, and Ivena Stupans in their chapter entitled *Health Service Organisation and Student Clinical Workplace Learning Opportunities* refer to the imperatives of practice (i.e. health-care practice) in shaping the experiences of students in health-care settings. They remind their readers that the primary purpose of health-care settings is the care of sick people, not a site for student placements. And, even in those health-care settings which are designated for clinical education, there are demands that arise from servicing the needs of students, sometimes with different institutional requirements, that cause complications and complexities which may not work in favour of supporting students' learning. Yet, in consideration of the specific circumstances of practice, the authors argue that because of the nature of health-care work, a strong disciplinary focus is likely to be that which sustains support for students, as health-care practitioners seek to balance a primary concern of health care with assisting students' learning. Moreover, the nature of the organisation of the particular health-care team shapes how the provision of student support is enacted. For instance, against what might be assumed within the university setting, there can be no guarantee that the person supervising the particular student is from their particular discipline. To make their point, the authors outline three different instances of clinical team profiles and how these profiles generated very distinct models of student support and supervision, and, therefore, experiences for students. These profiles include the composition of the health-care team, the diversity of disciplines, the kind of shift arrangements, and the kinds of activities that were generated by factors such as location. Beyond these differences in the organisation of health-care teams were also distinct perceptions of their roles and approaches to providing support.

In the final chapter – *Promoting Professional Learning: Individual and Institutional Practices and Imperatives* – Amanda Henderson draws out some deductions from the health-related studies which comprise a significant element of contributions within this volume. She refers to the importance of identifying the kinds of learning that need to occur and how these might best be organised across experiences in both the university and practice settings. In doing so, she also identifies particular curriculum pedagogic practices that can serve these purposes within health and related areas. The curriculum considerations include the staging and sequencing of practices and also take into consideration the importance of structuring these experiences in order to provide access to the kinds of knowledge that need to be learnt. In addition, considerations for pedagogic practices include students' intentions associated with their learning and how they will come to engage with the experiences provided for them. As mentioned above, in different ways, university students are now positioning themselves as being time jealous. That is, they carefully guard their time, as they negotiate busy lives in which the requirements for study are just one priority and in which demands on their time are high. Hence, they will not always engage actively in the activities they do not see as being directly relevant to their study goals (i.e. immediate requirements for successful completion of course components). The author refers to the importance of a range of strategies in university settings to engage students in considering and reflecting upon their experiences in practice settings, and highlights examples of these within particular contributions to this volume. In addition, she brings in the perspective from practice settings and highlights the key role that supervision in health-care practice settings can play in developing students' capacities, and again highlights examples of this role provided throughout the chapters. She concludes with a consideration of how organisational factors play out in what is possible to be afforded to students and promote their learning. For instance, she refers to different kinds of institutional arrangements that support the preparation of medical and nursing students, and the barriers that these create to bringing these two groups of students together to promote interprofessional learning. This is also used as an example of some of the difficult tensions that reside within institutional arrangements that seek to promote professional learning through university programmes. This chapter is particularly helpful and provides a useful conclusion to this publication in so far as it takes forward the diverse contributions and 'test bench' them from the perspective of a practitioner who has concerns about promoting professional learning in a health-care system. In doing so, it seeks to identify ways from the workplace perspective to secure effective integrations in order to realise productive outcomes from university programmes, the job-ready graduates that the health-care system so desperately needs.

Acknowledgements The author wishes to acknowledge the support provided by the Australian Learning and Teaching Council.

References

Australia. (2008). *A national internship scheme: Enhancing the skills and work-readiness of Australian university graduates*. Canberra, ACT: Universities Australia.

Billett, S. (2001). *Learning in the workplace: Strategies for effective practice*. Sydney: Allen and Unwin.

Billett, S. (2006). *Work, change and workers*. Dordrecht: Springer.

Billett, S. (2009). Realising the educational worth of integrating work experiences in higher education. *Studies in Higher Education, 34*(7), 827–843.

Boud, D., & Solomon, N. (Eds.). (2001). *Work-based learning: A new higher education?*. Buckingham: Open University Press.

Department of Innovation Universities and Skills. (2008). *Higher education at work: High skills: High value*.

Henderson, A., Twentyman, M., Heel, A., & Lloyd, B. (2006). Students' perception of the psychosocial clinical learning environment: An evaluation of the placement models. *Nurse Education Today, 26*(7), 564–571.

Jolly, B., & Macdonald, M. M. (1989). Education for practice: The role of practical experience in undergraduate and general clinical training. *Medical Education, 23*, 189–195.

Lomas, L. (1997). The decline of liberal education and the emergence of a new model of education and training. *Education + Training, 39*(3), 111–115.

Perkins, D., Jay, E., & Tishman, S. (1993). Beyond abilities: A dispositional theory of thinking. *Merrill-Palmer Quarterly, 39*(1), 1–21.

Stevenson, J. (1994). Vocational expertise. In J. Stevenson (Ed.), *Cognition at work* (pp. 7–34). Adelaide: National Centre for Vocational Education Research.

Chapter 2
Integrating Experiences in Workplace and University Settings: A Conceptual Perspective

Stephen Billett

2.1 Educational Purposes for Integrating Experiences in University and Practice Settings

Across many advanced industrial economies, there is a shift in the emphasis within higher education programmes away from the liberal arts and towards those that are primarily concerned with the preparation for specific occupations (Lomas, 1997). This change has led to descriptions, sometimes pejoratively, of universities now primarily being involved in 'higher vocational education'. With this shift in the focus of higher educational to more occupationally specific courses have also come expectations that university graduates will enjoy smooth transitions from their studies into professional practice and to function as effective practitioners (Department of Innovation Universities and Skills, 2008). That is, graduates are expected to have the capacities to engage immediately and effectively in the professional setting where they secure employment upon graduation. This expectation is a very exacting one. It suggests that university courses will need to prepare students not only in the canonical knowledge of the specific occupation (i.e. the procedural, conceptual and dispositional attributes expected of somebody practising that occupation) but also provide them with sufficient knowledge about the variations of that occupational practice that they will encounter when coming to practice it in particular workplace settings. This second set of requirements is often overlooked. However, both commonsensically and as has been demonstrated through research, the requirements for performing as a physiotherapist, nurse, doctor, engineer, journalist, etc. are far from uniform. Instead, the particular site of practice (i.e. workplace) will likely have particular requirements, purposes, clientele and other situational factors that shape what constitutes effective practice as a situated instance of occupational practice (Billett, 2001a). Of course, the actual situations where graduates will find employment are not always known or can even be predicted as students progress through their courses. Hence, preparing graduates for smooth transitions into practice is often

S. Billett (✉)
School of Education and Professional Studies, Griffith University, Brisbane,
QLD 4112, Australia
e-mail: s.billett@griffith.edu.au

S. Billett, A. Henderson (eds.), *Developing Learning Professionals*, Professional
and Practice-based Learning 7, DOI 10.1007/978-90-481-3937-8_2,
© Springer Science+Business Media B.V. 2011

premised on assisting them to know something about the variations in the occupational practice. Arguably, these kinds of outcomes are also what higher education students want and expect, employers increasingly demand and governments increasingly expect: highly and readily applicable learning outcomes. Yet, to get close to realising these kinds of outcomes across higher education programmes requires the organisation of learning experiences that can best develop these occupational capacities.

So, there are educational purposes associated with canonical and situational occupational requirements that need to be identified and experiences provided to assist students to secure working competence that meets these requirements. Yet, there are also other factors associated with the smooth transition into effective practice. One of these is the time it takes to develop competent performance, and how this can best be developed. For instance, it is often claimed that it takes a significant period of engagement in a domain of activity (e.g. an occupation) to become highly proficient or expert. Although the figure of 10 years is often used, some evidence suggests that it can be either more or less than a decade. More importantly, for the transition into practice there is a less specifiable period of time required to develop the range of capacities to engage effectively as a novice practitioner. Some studies suggest that this can be as little as 3 or 4 months, with others suggesting far longer periods (Ericsson, 2006). The duration of the time to become effectively operational will likely differ quite widely across occupations depending upon the massiveness of the knowledge to be learnt and the intricacies of procedures required for effective performance. What these considerations suggest is that there will need to be extensive periods of engagement in authentic practice during the preparatory educational programme to develop these operational capacities and a range of experiences. Hence, associated educational purposes will be about the adequacy of and duration of experiences in practice settings including the authenticity of those experiences, their duration and in what ways they engage students in active learning associated with the occupation. Ericsson (2006), in reviewing bodies of research into the processes of learning professional practice, including his own over 4 decades, concludes that the kind and duration of experiences are essential for the development of competent practice, but not wholly determinant. Instead, he notes the importance of deliberate practice in utilising fully and extending the contributions of those experiences. Ericsson has noted that a key indicator of the development of expert capacities is the degree by which the individual has engaged in effortful and focused deliberate practice. He provides examples of musicians whose private practice habits maximise and extend the provision of support they accessed from their teachers and other musicians. Consequently, his concept of learning through and for practice can be seen as being dualistic. On the one hand are the kinds of opportunities provided to support learners and experienced practitioners to engage in deliberate practice including their duration, and, on the other hand is the degree by which individuals elect to engage fully in that practice. Consequently, educational purposes for developing and promoting professional competence need to consider both the kinds of knowledge that need to be learnt, and the kind of experiences that are likely to be generative of that knowledge. All of this is leading to a growing interest in and an emphasis on work-integrated learning within higher education, albeit taking distinct forms across different disciplines and countries.

Yet, these kinds of purposes and processes are not wholly novel to higher education. They have been long exercised, for instance, by the North American co-op movement, through its provision of extensive periods of work placements (e.g. internships) (Grubb & Badway, 1998). Then, there is the long-standing arrangement of providing practicums in medicine, law, nursing, physiotherapy, etc. (e.g. Boud & Solomon, 2001) that has been well accepted within these programmes and long since been seen as being essential for the development of these occupations. However, while these practice-based experiences have long been included in the curriculum, the increased emphasis on providing such experiences and integrating them within the overall course curriculum and the increased expectations associated with generating competent practitioners suggest the need to understand and organise these experiences more fully.

A starting point here is to identify the forms and kinds of knowledge required for practice so that considerations about how the university and practice settings can contribute to this knowledge being learnt by students. This consideration comprises understanding the occupational domain-specific conceptual, procedural and dispositional forms of knowledge, including the kinds of attributes that that professional practitioners need to exercise: diligence, care, precision, etc. Central to the learning of this knowledge and its effective exercise and development across working life are individuals exercising their agency in learning about, performing and monitoring their work and ongoing learning.

In all, educational processes are supposed to be intentional, guided by purposes that are considered, and informed by the kinds of goals to be achieved and the kinds of learning that are supposed to arise from them. Hence, it is necessary to understand the forms of knowledge that are the focus of these educational purposes and then, the means by which these purposes are realised in assisting students' learning.

2.1.1 Conceptual, Procedural, Dispositional Knowledge: Canonical Forms and Situational Versus Personal Attributes

Much consideration has been given to the kinds of knowledge that underpins human performance. Indeed, this was a key project for the cognitive movement of the last 3 decades. The findings have informed concepts about and have become a key focus for educational processes. One key contribution of this work has been to go beyond just valuing conceptual knowledge. Indeed, the long-standing privileging of conceptual knowledge has done much to elevate the status of this form of knowledge as being the most worthwhile. It seems that the legacy of a hierarchy of knowledge established in ancient Greece by Aristotle still plays out in contemporary educational discourses. That is, learning about concepts is seen to be privileged over the capacities (i.e. procedures) to undertake tasks. The origins of such a hierarchy are easy to explain, being premised upon a division of labour in which freeborn male Greek citizens were not supposed to engage in any form of occupation, except certain elite versions (military), and where the majority of work was seen to be procedural and not worthy of gainful pursuits by freeborn Greek citizens. Since then there has been a privileging of concepts over procedural capacities, most prominently and erroneously presented as the theory and practice divide. Such privileging was questioned by Ryle (1949) who suggested that beyond knowing about things – 'knowing that' – there was also the ghost within the machine that realised outcomes – 'know-how'. This contribution energised a consideration of procedural capacities and questioned its lowly standing against conceptual attributes. Indeed, across 3 decades of focused inquiry into what constitutes expert performance, largely within cognitive psychology, but not restricted to it, there has been developed a more comprehensive understanding of the kinds of knowledge required for effective occupational practice (i.e. expertise) (Chi, Feltovich, & Glaser, 1981; Chi, Glaser, & Farr, 1982; K A Ericsson & Lehmann, 1996; Glaser, 1989; Larkin, McDermott, Simon, & Simon, 1980), and an emphasis on the strategic qualities of higher orders of procedural knowledge. This inquiry sought to identify the kinds of qualities that distinguished experts from novices to understand how the latter could best progress to the former, in order to inform both the goals for and processes of that development. During this period of intense investigation it became apparent that considerations of concepts and procedures in themselves were also inadequate as this classification fails to adequately account for personal attitudes, interests and values (Perkins, Jay, & Tishman, 1993). Hence, a consideration of the dispositions that shape the engagement with and enactment of conceptual and procedural knowledge was included in accounts describing the attributes of affect. However, this occupational knowledge is more than 'techne' – technical capacity; it is far broader and more encompassing. There is the need to 'generate and evaluate skilled performance as technical tasks become complex and as situations and processes change, reason and solve technical problems, be strategic, innovate and adapt' (Stevenson, 1994, p. 9). Moreover, professionals also need critical insights and to be reflexive in how they apply what they know as requirements for work change or are shaped by particular situational requirements that cause decisions to be made about how to progress amongst a range of possible options.

Drawing these contributions together in a classification system which can be used to inform educational purposes and processes, it seems that effective occupational performance relies upon three forms of interrelated knowledge. These are as follows:

- Domain-specific conceptual knowledge – 'knowing that' (Ryle, 1949) (i.e. concepts, facts, propositions – surface to deep, e.g. Glaser, 1989).
- Domain-specific procedural knowledge – 'knowing how' (Ryle, 1949) (i.e. specific to strategic procedures, e.g. Anderson, 1993).
- Dispositional knowledge – 'knowing for' (i.e. values, attitudes) related to both canonical and instances of practice (e.g. Perkins et al., 1993), includes criticality (e.g. Mezirow, 1981).

These forms of knowledge pertain to particular domains of activity (e.g. an occupation), rather than being generalisable capacities, and therefore performance premised on them is largely specific to that domain of activity. Each of these forms of domain-specific knowledge has its own qualities (e.g. specific and strategic procedures, factual to complex conceptual premises) that have arisen through history, and that have cultural relevance (i.e. respond to cultural needs) and situational pertinence (i.e. respond to the requirements of particular situations). Knowledge that has these qualities is likely to be developed by individuals through opportunities to engage in and construct personal, and possibly idiosyncratic, domains of the occupational knowledge. Indeed, there seems to be at least three levels of domain-specific knowledge (Scribner, 1984). First, there is the canonical knowledge of the occupation, comprising what those practising this occupation would be expected to know. It is this domain of activity that is often the focus of professional registration, occupational standards and national curriculum development exercises. Indeed, this is the kind of knowledge often attempted to be stated as occupational standards and captured as statements for performance and curriculum content and outcomes. Yet, while this canonical occupational knowledge is important and needs to be learnt, and is often the focus of educational efforts, occupational performance is also shaped by situational factors that constitute the requirements for actual performance in practice.

Consequently, and second, there is the manifestation of the requirements where the occupation is practised: the knowledge required for a particular instance of practice, because canonical performance requirements alone would be insufficient to inform practice in specific circumstances. Instead, it is necessary for the requirements of the situation or setting to be acknowledged, because practice occurs and is judged in particular circumstances. In this way, it is only when that occupational knowledge is utilised in a particular setting, at a particular point in time and in responding to particular work tasks that it is actually manifested as practice. It is in these situations where individuals come to engage with, learn about and practice the particular occupation. Also, here, as noted, is where judgements are made about performance. Importantly, there is no such thing as an occupational expert per se. These can only be made in the circumstances where that practice is enacted and where it is possible to make judgements about the efficacy and elegance or otherwise of that practice.

Third, is the personally constructed domain of occupational knowledge that arises ontogenetically (i.e. throughout individuals' life history). That is, individuals construct their own accounts of the occupational practice through engagement with it and learn about it in educational programmes and other kinds of experiences. Yet, that process of construction is not merely the transfer of knowledge osmosis like from the world outside the individuals into them. Instead, the process is interpsychological: arising through the relations that comprise individuals' construal and construction of what they encounter in the world beyond themselves. Consequently, rather than being taught, to become effective practitioners, individuals need to construct the domain-specific procedural, conceptual (Glaser, 1984) and dispositional (Perkins et al., 1993) capacities required for the occupational practice, at both the canonical level and in the circumstances in which they practice. That is, they need to learn the domain-specific procedures, concepts and values required to be a doctor, hairdresser, plumber, vacuum-cleaner salesperson or lighthouse keeper, and also the particular set of concepts, procedures and dispositions that are required for effective practice in the particular circumstances in which doctoring, hairdressing, plumbing, vacuum-cleaner selling and lighthouse keeping are practised (Billett, 2001a). Yet, these forms of knowledge are those required to be accessed and constructed by individuals who are seeking to learn them. Consequently, experiences provided for students have to include those that can assist them to access and construct the knowledge required for a smooth transition from educational institution into practice, and then to effective operational roles and onto becoming an occupational expert. To elaborate these forms of knowledge a little more the following descriptions are provided.

Conceptual or declarative knowledge comprises concepts, fact, propositions and the richly interlinked associations among them. This form of knowledge can be spoken about and written down. Hence, this knowledge is sometimes termed as 'declarative' (Anderson, 1982; Glaser, 1984): it can be declared. Much of this knowledge is representable in books, texts and other forms of media or artefacts, although often at the lower levels of facts, propositions and, with more difficulty, linked associations. It has been proposed that the progression of the complex conceptual development tends to move from understanding basic factual knowledge through to propositions and associations between conceptual knowledge (Anderson, 1982), which is sometimes described as conceptual understandings. However, rather than being ponderous and massive, that is knowing a lot, deep conceptual knowledge is premised on understanding the relations between sets of concepts and propositions of this kind (Groen & Patel, 1988). It is this depth, in terms of links and associations, which arises from long-term engagement and different kinds of episodes within in a particular domain of activity and a variety of experiences. However, as Ericsson (2006) advises, while extensive experience is a necessary quality for developing the conceptual knowledge it is not sufficient. In addition, there has to be ways in which engagements by learners can be assisted to make links and associations among concepts in order for that kind of level of development to arise. Much of this has to come from the learner.

Procedural knowledge is that which we use to do things, yet which cannot be easily declared or represented, because much of it is rendered tacit in its construction (Anderson, 1982; Shuell, 1990). More than referring to physical movement, as in psychomotor capacities, procedures also refer to the processes of thinking and acting (i.e. cognition). That is, the very processes of engaging concepts and identifying associations, amongst many others, such as reading this text, arise from the use of procedures. In this way, much of procedural knowledge is wholly unobservable, which frustrates those who seek to measure and calibrate it. Sometimes, this leads to it being simply ignored. Indeed, the ghost in the machine (Ryle, 1949) is not accounted for in behavioural explanations of human performance. As noted, procedural knowledge is often required to be engaged with and practised for its development to occur. Indeed, the progression from specific procedures through to strategic procedural knowledge is seen as a process of rehearsing specific procedures in ways that remove the need for conscious memory to be enacted in their deployment, permitting that conscious memory to focus on more strategic issues (Anderson, 1982). Then, through engaging in an extensive array of episodes of knowledge use which are also monitored and critically appraised, effective strategic procedural knowledge arise, albeit within the domain of activities. Hence, this development, at all levels, likely arises from the opportunity to participate in a range of activities and interludes associated with the particular domain of activity for which the procedures are being developed. At one level, the rehearsal of specific procedures (i.e. practise) permits them to be enacted without recourse to conscious thought. This capacity is important because it allows individuals to use their conscious memory to perform other or more strategic aspects of tasks while specific procedures are being enacted. At another level, the repertoire of experiences that individuals access and understand leads to the ability to predict and evaluate performance, and this also arises through opportunities to practise. Again, here Ericsson (2006) would advise that deliberate practice is essential. This is likely to be no more so than as a development of procedural knowledge encompasses its strategic forms, because its development is so effortful and will not arise without this kind of intentional rehearsal.

Dispositional knowledge comprises interests and beliefs, which not only energise the use and development of concepts and procedures (Perkins et al., 1993), but also shape the direction, intensity, and degree of their enactment (Billett, 2008b). Indeed, given the key role that humans play in their own learning and development, the purposes for, and intentionality and intensity by which they engage in construing and constructing knowledge is central to the quality of their learning. All of these processes are underpinned by dispositions. Within a personal domain, dispositions are likely developed through individuals' beliefs and are negotiated through their encounters with particular experiences. Yet, they also exist as social facts. That is, there are particular dispositions associated with occupations that become central to their enactment. The care and diligence of the accountant or auditor, the caution of an airline pilot, the sympathy of a human care worker and the ethical conduct of a counsellor are but some examples here. Yet, such dispositional prescriptions are inert and stand as propositions only until they are applied in practice. It is through the agency of the individual in exercising care and diligence when accounting, cautiousness and what constitutes it as a pilot, and sympathetic engagement with different kinds of people that these dispositions become personal occupational attributes.

What has been proposed above is that the interrelated forms of knowledge referred to above have canonical, situational and personal manifestations. Yet, beyond occupationally specific domains of knowledge are also attributes that play across these three manifestations. One which concerns us particularly here is workers' conduct and agency. It is perhaps reasonable to expect both at the canonical and situational level that workers are responsible for engaging in and monitoring their work and performance, and being proactive in continuing to learn more about that practice. Moreover, for work nominated as being 'professional', there is a heightened expectation of self-directedness in terms of enacting, monitoring and extending personal competence. This particular attribute is important here because not only is it a quality required of professional workers, but it is also essential to the processes of learning about that occupation and maintaining competence across working life. As discussed below, in terms of initial learning and experiences provided across the two settings and the integration of those experiences (i.e. comprehension and reconciliation), these are tasks that learners undertake, because it is they who engage in and negotiate their experiences and learning across both the practice and educational settings. Their engagement with these experiences and deliberate practice are central to the quality of their initial and ongoing learning.

Moreover, the three forms of knowledge described above are richly interconnected and interdependent in their manifestation, development and enactment. This very connectedness and interdependence arises through episodes of practice in which these forms of knowledge are deployed and developed together when enacting domain-specific activities (Billett, 2001b). Indeed, cognitive theorists (e.g. Anderson, 1982) view the development of these forms of knowledge arising interdependently through which individuals construe and construct experiences (i.e. conceptual to procedural development). It is through these episodes of practice that certainty about performance is developed, procedures automated and dispositions tested. So, not only does expertise take time and extensive repertoires of experience to develop and hone (Anderson, 1982), but it is also shaped through particular episodes of experiences that are afforded by the situated instances of practice in which individuals engage and how they make sense of those experiences.

The importance of what has been proposed above is that these forms of knowledge and their distinct manifestations stand as being the key goals that comprise the purposes of educational processes concerned with developing occupational specific competence. Of course, the development of these capacities only commences within university courses preparing students for their selected occupation. It continues and is ongoing across professionals' working lives. Nevertheless, it behoves those who organise learning experiences (i.e. the curriculum) within higher education institutions to try and provide particular interventions that can secure particular kinds of learning (i.e. pedagogy) in order to understand something of the forms of knowledge to be learnt and consider how best that might occur. Also, from all that has been proposed above, in terms of the construction of personal domains of knowledge, considerations of engagement and deliberate practice, it is necessary to consider the importance of developing students as agentic learners.

2.1.2 Agency of Learners

Given the central role of learners in construing and constructing knowledge from what they experience and shaping the ways in which these processes occur, it is also important to emphasise the salience of students as agentic learners; that is as active, directed and intentional learners. Indeed, they are the very kind which Ericsson (2006) refers to as engaging in deliberate practice, albeit on their own and often in self-directed ways. Certainly, it is students who participate in, negotiate, and learn in and across both practice and university settings. Ultimately, they are the meaning makers who will negotiate learning across these settings, not their teachers, tutors or mentors, although the latter can do much to support that learning. As already noted, the process of students' learning is ongoing and ubiquitous, yet shaped by what students encounter in educational institutions and practice settings and how they construe, construct, and engage with what is afforded them. Therefore, active engagement and learning by university students is a likely pre-requisite for the kinds of higher order learning required for the principle-based and codified forms of occupational knowledge that underpin professional work. Moreover, this kind of engagement is applicable for many, if not most, forms of occupational practice, and not only for the top-end professionals (e.g. law and medicine). Indeed, the expectation for practitioners whose occupation carries the moniker of 'professions' is for them to be self-directed in the learning to maintain the currency of the professional practice: to profess. The point here is that the very qualities needed to be an effective student in higher education – a proactive and agentic learner – are those required for effective professional practice. In essence, the agentic qualities of learners are essential for effective professional practice, yet also for the initial and ongoing learning associated with that practice. Consequently, more than attempting to organise experiences for students in educational institutions and workplace settings to learn the conceptual, procedural and dispositional knowledge at both the canonical and situational level, there is a need to focus on preparing students to be agentic learners, as part of their professional preparation. It is these capacities that will also assist their transition to practice and maintaining effective practice across their working lives.

Having discussed the kinds of educational purposes that are required for developing effective occupational practice, and offered a classification of both domains of knowledge and forms of knowledge that need to be learnt, it is therefore appropriate now to consider how experiences in both university and practice settings can be used for promoting students' learning of this knowledge.

2.2 Conceptions of Contributions from Both Settings: Beyond the Theory-Practice Divide

It has been long suggested that different learning outcomes arise for students from experiences in practice and educational settings. One of the most common and enduring differences is that educational institutions are generative of theory, and experiences in workplaces lead to the development of the procedural capacities required to practice. Indeed, it is often suggested that conceptual knowledge arises through participation in university-type experiences and procedural emerged through engagement in practice settings. Clearly this is a simple and erroneous proposition as has been argued above. Components of all three forms of knowledge (i.e. conceptual, procedural and dispositional) can be accessed in each setting, because they provide access to and opportunities for their learning through the kinds of activities and interactions that they provide. There is no necessarily privileging of the kinds of knowledge that can be learnt in each of these settings. That is, robust or transferable knowledge is as likely to arise through experiences in practice settings and educational institutions (Rogoff & Lave, 1984). However, the activities and interactions afforded by each of these are likely to be generative of particular kinds of learning.

Indeed, the kinds of activities in which individuals engage shape their learning or, as Rogoff and Lave (1984, p. v) suggest, 'activity structures cognition'. This structuring appears to occur as follows. When humans engage with goal-directed activities they deploy and engage their knowledge in undertaking the task. This permits us to enact a task, monitor its progress and consequences, modify approaches and evaluate the outcomes of these various stages. Not only is knowledge deployed during engagement in these goal-directed activities, but also there are legacies arising from their enactment. Those legacies can comprise the refining of what we know, or transformation of that knowledge. Moreover, the conduct of goal-directed activities is also shaped by the social and physical context in which they occur, which often provides clues and cues about how to proceed, some goals for performance and the capacity to monitor progress (Lave, Murtaugh, & de la Roche, 1984). When these activities are undertaken in circumstances which are similar, the same or at least analogous to those in which the learnt knowledge is to be applied, the legacies are likely to be more applicable than when they occur in circumstances which are apparently remote from those in which the knowledge is to be applied. Therefore, providing access to activities and interactions that are authentic in terms of the performances required to be learnt and practised becomes essential for learning effective practice. Currently, many of higher education students' learning experiences are shaped by universities' institutional practices and physical and social settings, which are distinct from professional practice. While substitute experiences (e.g. moot courts and mock hospital wards) are useful in providing a benign environment in which to develop initial capacities, they do not provide access to the array of clues and cues, some goals and ultimately the access to the kinds of dispositional, procedural and conceptual contributions that are available in authentic professional practice (Billett, 2001a). So the 'canonical' professional concepts, procedures and dispositions that might be learnt in university settings need augmenting by understandings, procedures and sentiments learnt through experiences in authentic instances of professional practice: practice-based experiences. Authentic practice (i.e. workplace) experiences can make particular and potent contributions to students' learning (Billett, 2001b), and likely do so in ways that provide access to activities and interactions, expert practitioners in ways simply unavailable in university settings.

Moreover, engaging in authentic instances of practice provides the basis to understand some of the variations of professional practice, thereby making what has been learnt in university courses more likely applicable to diverse instances and requirements of practice that graduates will encounter as they move into paid employment. Early views of human performance suggested that adaptability was premised on generally applicable capacities (Bartlett, 1958) and, then, on the possession of domain-specific knowledge and the capacity to manipulate it (Ericsson & Smith,

1991). However, more recently, understanding the specific and situational bases for performance to be enacted has been emphasised (e.g. Billett, 2001a; Brown, Collins, & Duguid, 1989; Engestrom & Middleton, 1996). Hence, the development of adaptability and the competence required for practice might well be found in utilising a range of these experiences within the university setting. This capacity is central to the expectation that graduates will be able to move smoothly into effective occupational practice, because without understanding some of the variations of how the canonical knowledge of the occupation is applied, graduates as new employees might experience dissonance between what they know and what they experience. As discussed below, there are a number of ways in which students' understanding of some of the variations of these practices can be generated that does not necessarily involve them in engaging in a broad array of experiences themselves. However, it is important that their conceptions and responses are informed by considering their occupational practice as being diverse rather than unitary.

While much of the discussion above has focused on the contributions arising from practice settings there is much that experiences within university settings can contribute to effective professional preparation. Studies into what and how people learn through practice have identified the importance of assisting learners develop understanding, dispositions and procedures in environments and through experiences which are best able to achieve these goals. Certainly, specific aspects of knowledge about practice may be inaccessible or unavailable in workplace settings because it is neither experienced nor accessible. For instance, in one study it was found that hairdressers understanding of the structure of hair were quite limited and, where extensive, was the product of engaged classroom experiences. Moreover, the increased use of symbolic knowledge within the array of technical-derived activities within contemporary workplaces (Billett, 2006) makes this form of knowledge hard to learn through practice because it is often not easy to access by learners). Hence, this form of knowledge might best be developed through appropriate pedagogic experiences in circumstances where that knowledge can be made more accessible. One clear contribution which can be perhaps best established in the university setting is the means for students to become effective self-directed and agentic learners, not only for their initial preparation, but also for their professional lives. That is, students need to intentionally develop, through their engagement within practicum environments, effective personal epistemologies that will support the initial and ongoing learning required for competent professional practice. Hence, there is a need for educators to engage with students to assist them to become intentionally active learners and selecting appropriate teaching and learning approaches to secure this outcome, including utilising and integrating practice-based experiences (e.g. Chapter 4, this volume).

Given the case made above that both kinds of settings make particular contributions to students' occupational preparation and ongoing development in their professional work, it follows that the bringing together these two sets of contributions and effectively integrating them becomes an important curriculum and pedagogic priority for higher education. Yet, before curriculum means and pedagogic practices can be organised and enacted effectively, it is important to understand what constitutes such integrations, and how best they can be realised productively. In the next section, a view about what constitutes integrations is proposed.

2.2.1 Constituting Integration

As foreshadowed in Chapter 1 and noted above, in a number of countries, the integration of students' learning experiences across educational and practice settings is becoming of growing interest within higher education institutions and governments. Following this, much effort and many resources are being now expended, seemingly across all disciplines, to secure practice-based experiences for university students. However, beyond securing student access to experiences in practice settings, there is also the need for the learning arising from these experiences to be effectively integrated into the students' overall curriculum. This goal necessitates making explicit the links between what is learnt through experiences in both settings, and then finding ways to integrate those contributions. It is unlikely that students will realise smooth transitions and effective practice without their making links between the learning arising for them from experiences in both settings. Also, the utilisation of both institutional resources by universities and practice settings, as well as personal investments by students, will not be optimised unless the contributions to students' learning in both settings are effectively engaged and integrated.

Yet, despite their importance, there are few satisfactory explanatory accounts about what constitutes such integrations, and how they might be best realised in higher education (Eames & Coll, 2010). This gap makes difficult the process of selecting the kinds of curriculum and pedagogic practices that are appropriate to secure these integrations, and for particular educational purposes (Grollman & Tutschner, 2006; Stenstrom et al., 2006). Drawing on existing conceptions and theories of learning, there are a number of ways in which the integration of learning experiences across academic and practice settings might be considered and realised. Commonly used terms such as the transfer of knowledge and adaptability of learning provide some bases from cognitive theory to explain the integration process. Proposed here is the idea of these integrations comprising a dual process described as a socio-personal process.

A helpful starting point for conceptualising the integration of learning experiences is the assumptions that learning arises through people's experiences and that learning is nothing other than change within individuals. That is, and building upon what has been advanced above, the ongoing interaction between people and the social and physical world constitutes individuals' experiences comprising both what is suggested to them, on the one hand, and how they construe those experiences and change as a result of those experiences, on the other (Billett, 2008a). Moreover, the change or learning that arises can comprise experiences that provide for the verification, reinforcement and further honing of what individuals already know, can do or value. These kinds of conceptual, procedural and dispositional learning arise continually through engagement in activities or interactions which are familiar to or routine for us (Lee & Roth, 2005). Alternatively, and by degree, this change can also involve new understandings, beliefs and ways of doing things that may arise through engagement in experiences that are novel or transformational for individuals. Both kinds of experiences have the capacity to extend individuals' knowledge in ways that simply would not have been possible had they not had that kind of experience. However, novel experiences can also be overwhelming, and cause dissonance in an unhelpful and unsatisfactory way. Hence, humans' experiences and their learning are one and the same, because they comprise the same cognitive process.

Within such a view, what is often referred to as transfer or adaptability is held to be consonant with routine experiences comprising 'near' transfer and with non-routine experiences comprising 'far' transfer (Voss, 1987). In all of these differently labelled processes, there are common features of individuals experiencing something, aligning and reconciling what has been experienced with what they know and then reinforcing, honing or transforming their knowing. However, such experiences and learning (i.e. experiencing) are person dependent because what constitutes the experience and the learning that arises from it is shaped by how individuals construe and construct their experience based on earlier or pre-mediate experiences (Valsiner & van der Veer, 2000). It is the processes of individuals' linking and reconciling experiences that is most helpful in explaining what might constitute integrations between academic and practical settings. Well established principally within, but not restricted to, psychological thought is the claim that individuals will attempt and be successful, by degree, in seeking to link what they know with what they experience, and then attempt to reconcile any differences that emerge. For instance, most famously, Piaget (1968) referred to individuals seeking to overcome disequilibrium by reconciling what they know with what they experience, thereby securing equilibrium. More recent constructivist accounts such as those of Van Lehn (1989) and von Glasersfeld (1987) refer to a similar phenomenon that they call the process of maintaining viability. That is, individuals seeking to make what they experience viable in terms of what they already know. Similarly, the social phenomenologist Schutz (1970) refers to typification – the process in which new experiences are ordered on the basis of how individuals have come to typify what they know. Then, quite analogously, the sociologist Giddens (1991) refers to individuals seeking ontological security: striving to make sense of what they encounter in the social world. These different accounts are in many ways quite consistent and premised on the idea that humans are active meaning makers and constructors of their knowledge that arises through what they experience, and that they are also active in seeking to reconcile what they experience with what they know, or want to know. All these accounts refer to individuals' processes of making links or associations between what they know and engaging in a process of reconciliation with what they experience.

The processes required for integrating experiences in both academic and practice settings seem consonant with what has been described in these conceptual accounts of learning (e.g. securing equilibrium, viability, typification and subjectification). The processes of securing those integrations they might be described as making associations and reconciliations between the contributions of two settings. The act of integrating experiences comprises a negotiation between individuals' cognitive experience (Valsiner, 2000) (i.e. what they know and how they experience the world) and what is suggested to them through the norms and forms of the physical and social world that they encounter. Therefore, explaining the processes of integration of experiences in academic and practice settings requires accounting for the active process by students of making associations and realising reconciliations between what they know and experience. In this way, the process of linking and reconciling experiences in different settings, referred to here to as integration, seemingly comprises a commonplace process of human meaning-making. So, on their own terms, there is nothing particularly unusual about the cognitive processes that underpin the process of integrating experiences across different settings. However, as with all important processes of development they are effortful and often require guidance and support.

Indeed, because of the inherently personal character of these integrations, it is important that the process that supports them be considered in greater detail. To begin with, while the various accounts of personal meaning-making above emphasise the agency of the individual in constructing that meaning, much less is advanced about how they will actually enact this process. That is, the degree of intentionality and effort with which individuals engage in the processes of linking and reconciliation may not always be directed towards the intended educational outcomes. Clearly, individuals have to be selective about what they engage with because the demands and suggestions of the social world are such that individuals have to rebuff the majority of what is suggested to them (Valsiner, 1998) to maintain their equilibrium/viability/typification/subjectification. Indeed, as Baldwin (1894) identified much earlier, individuals' engagement with the world beyond them is undertaken selectively. Therefore, ultimately, it is individuals that direct their efforts and intentionality in the process of integrating experiences through linking and reconciliation. In the first instance, then, as learners are faced with different settings for learning, they might need to be guided in the ways they should exercise their agency and the purposes of the different experiences. As well, in many higher education courses, students' engagement in the intense process of learning occupational tasks, often occur over short periods of time, hence reconciliations are often formative and, thus, are likely to be, by degree, tentative, partial, incomplete and immature. Consequently, there may need to be some forms of assistance provided to students to guide and direct their integration. Therefore, even within a process which is inherently person dependent, purposeful integrations may not be wholly effective without some guidance and support. In sum, these integrations appear as a process of making links between sets of experiences and reconciling them in ways that are likely to be personally constructed, albeit negotiated with the social contributions.

The particular emphasis on students negotiating learning arising through activities and interactions in two distinct social settings (i.e. educational and practice) suggests a need to include a consideration of physical and social settings, as well as cognitive processes within accounts which can explain integrations and how they might best progress.

2.2.2 Three Accounts of Integrations

From the discussions above arise three accounts of what constitutes integrations. These comprise one focused on settings (i.e. a situational account), the second on individual constructions (i.e. personal constructivist account) and a third that seeks to reconcile the first two conceptions (i.e. a socio-personal account). The third of these – the socio-personal account – is held to provide the most comprehensive account of what constitutes such integrations and is advanced here. Yet, each of these three accounts is worth briefly discussing, as the first two inform the third.

The first of these, the situational account, emphasises the characteristics and potential contributions of the activities and interactions provided by both the education and practice settings. Central here is accounting for students' learning arising from both of these kinds of settings, and how they might be reconciled. That is, curriculum developers would identify how each setting can contribute to realising the particular educational purposes and then construct the curriculum and pedagogic means to utilise and integrate those contributions productively. In this approach, the settings are viewed as objective entities that have particular qualities and are able to provide students with access to particular forms of knowledge. That is, they provide access to specific kinds of conceptual, procedural and dispositional knowledge through affording particular kinds of activities and interactions. Hence, by participating in both of these settings students will have access to different contributions and will be able to augment these experiences through bringing both sets of learning together.

The second – personal constructivist account – focuses on students as active constructors of their knowledge in each setting and as the central focus in the task of integrating what has been experienced (and learnt) in both settings. In this account, the learners' process of 'experiencing' is emphasised and is viewed in terms of how they subjectively construe and construct knowledge from what they experience in and across the two settings. Here, there is a strong privileging of the phenomenological bases of learning as articulated above by what Schutz (1970) proposes. This account of integration emphasises the active process of appropriation (i.e. learners making some of what they experience their own) that arises through individuals' engagement with the two different social and physical settings. Yet, this view emphasises the process of meaning-making as being one which privileges individuals' construction of what they experience, more than the strength of the social suggestion which was advanced in the first account. Clearly, the strength and the contributions of the social setting will vary both in terms of its projection and its attraction to learners.

The third – socio-personal account – comprises a combination of both of these approaches. It acknowledges the duality and interdependence of the contributions of the settings and how individuals construe what is learnt: a socio-personal conception of the integration of these experiences. Here, the explanation of integration includes a consideration of what each of the environments can potentially does and should afford students. Moreover, it also accommodates how students can and should engage in, learn through and integrate these experiences, albeit in personally distinct ways. That is, rather than seeing either the social setting or the personal construction as being wholly dominant, both sets of contributions are interdependent, yet relational. They are interdependent because the social suggestion is nothing more than an invitation that requires individuals to engage with and take up what is being afforded them. Yet, the knowledge required to be learnt by students resides within the social and physical world with which learners must engage. Nevertheless, how they engage with it is relational on a number of bases. At one level, it is about individuals' level of knowledge and knowing that will shape how and to what purpose they engage with the social and physical world. This varies across learners. Then, there are the quite distinct personal histories or ontogenies with which individuals engage and which are generative of particular constructions and valuing of knowledge and institutions, etc. It is these ontogenies that ultimately shape how individuals make sense of what they experience. The integration of different kinds of experiences is shaped by individuals' processes of construal and construction that are often premised upon what they have already experienced – pre-mediately, albeit in person-dependent ways. Thus, the linking of experiences from university and practice settings is likely to be quite distinct across a cohort of students. For instance, experienced enrolled nurses entering an undergraduate nursing degree will likely have very different bases for construing and constructing knowledge about nursing (their personal experience) from what they experience in the university programme, than a school leaver without clinical experience (Newton, Billett, Jolly, & Ockerby, 2009). Moreover, how they each will come to link and reconcile what has been experienced and learnt is also likely to be person dependent by degree. So, while there may well be intents on the part of the educational programme for the linking and reconciliation of two different sets of experiences, these will always be negotiated in part by individuals.

Across all of this discussion about integrations, the need for curriculum and pedagogy to provide experiences in both kinds of settings and find ways of engaging and guiding learners in the construction of knowledge is strongly emphasised.

2.3 Towards Effective Integration: Pedagogy and Curriculum

In the discussions above, a number of principles emerge that are important for informing curriculum and pedagogy. First, it is through students' engagement in distinct kinds of activities and interactions in both practice and educational settings that learning for professional practice progresses. This arises through the processes of accessing and appropriating the forms of knowledge that are required for both canonical and situational levels of practice. Moreover, second, it is finding ways of associating and reconciling those different experiences in ways that are directed towards securing the knowledge required for professional practice that becomes the key organising principle for both curriculum and pedagogy. Third, it is not sufficient for pedagogy and curriculum to focus only on the provision of experiences; there needs to be strong emphases on how and what students experience. With these principles briefly articulated, some considerations for curriculum and pedagogy to integrate experiences across education and practice settings are now advanced in conclusion.

2.3.1 Considerations for Curriculum

A key consideration for curriculum is the organisation of experiences and in what sequences they should be provided for students. This consideration includes at what point practice-based experiences should be provided. In some programmes, these experiences are reserved for the final year or years. In these circumstances it is held that students require a range of competences before coming to engage in those experiences. However, other views suggest that practice-based experiences should occur from the beginning of the educational programme, and should be organised to meet specific learning goals and incrementally engage students in more demanding practice roles. So, for instance, it might be argued that nursing, medical and physiotherapy students should engage in practice experiences early in their programmes to understand the context of that practice and the kinds of work tasks that it involves, and to familiarise themselves with particular practice requirements. These roles might be largely observational or wholly assisting others. Then, subsequently, they might engage in programmes which position them to engage in a restricted set of productive work tasks, guided by more expert practitioner, before moving through into taking increasing responsibility and more complex work roles in subsequent practice experiences. Organisationally, it might be argued that both doctors and nurses should commence their practical experience in working as hospital orderlies, then, for doctors, by working as nurses, and then moving to their own practice. Similarly, student teachers might work as and with teacher aides, before going on to work with teachers. These kind of experiences may assist novices understand their particular occupation and its relationship to others, and upon what foundations their work builds. In all, the kind of sequencing needs to be mindful of curriculum as pathways in which experiences are provided that permit both new experiences and an opportunity to practice, refine and hone what has already been learnt. That is, combinations of familiar and new experiences should comprise these practicum experiences.

The organisation of these experiences includes a consideration of time allocated to experiences in both settings and how the practice-based experiences might be aligned with particular sets of educational intents that are inherent within the student programmes. That is, sequencing ought to align the provision of experiences within the educational setting with what students will engage within the practice settings. In all this, it will be likely that the educational institution and educators will need to take leadership in terms of organising and sequencing experience, because they most likely have the educational expertise to organise, monitor and evaluate these experiences. Of course, all of this should progress with considerations borne out of what constitutes the most likely pathway through which novice practitioners will come to know and learn that practice, realise the kind of domain-specific knowledge required to practice the occupation, and come to know something of the variations of that practice. For instance, curriculum and pedagogic processes that assist students share and appraise their experiences in different practice settings may well be helpful in developing robust knowledge associated with a particular occupation.

2.3.2 Considerations for Pedagogy

Essentially, pedagogy comprises the actions taken by others to enrich learning experiences. In this case, the concern is to assist, utilise and integrate the experiences and learning that is occurring in both settings. At the same time, there is a concern to develop students as agentic learners as they will need such qualities to learn effectively and integrate that learning across both settings, practice autonomously and develop further throughout their working lives.

As proposed elsewhere (Billett, 2009), an important consideration is for preparing students prior to their practice-based experiences, finding ways of supporting enjoying those experiences and then utilising and sharing the learning when they return from those experiences. There are particular educational purposes behind interventions in each of these three phases. Preparation needs to go beyond developing the conceptual and procedural capacities required to perform certain tasks, and needs to expand to ensuring that the learners are going to engage in active processes of learning through which they will maximise their experiences and find ways of integrating them. So, pedagogic activities here will be about establishing goals and processes for active learning, as well as advising about workplace requirements and potential difficulties that students may need to negotiate or resolve. Likely, processes that place students in a responsible and leaderly role, rather than those that are teacherly, would be the most successful. As reported elsewhere in this text, the use of focus groups, learning circles and discussion groups all are important in engaging students in preparing for and reflecting upon their experiences. In addition, considerations about the sharing of experiences in ways which assist students develop understandings about the different ways in which the professional practice is enacted is an important educational goal. It seems likely that it is these kinds of critical and shared reflections that are important for understanding how variations of practice occur and different approaches that can be used to secure particular outcomes, given access to particular kinds of resources, problems or contexts. Hence, there may be quite different kinds of pedagogic interventions prior to students engaging in practicum work: supporting them throughout and re-engaging with them on their return. Yet, within all this, a key concern is to provide guidance to students and also for them to engage in self-directed and reflective practice in which they play key roles in the process of identifying associations and reconciling what they have experienced in both the educational and practice settings. It is this quality that would not only be central to their reconciliation of experiences across both academic and practice settings, but will also prepare them for effective practice and their ongoing development across working lives.

Acknowledgements The author wishes to acknowledge the support provided by the Australian Learning and Teaching Council.

References

Anderson, J. R. (1982). Acquisition of cognitive skill. *Psychological Review, 89*(4), 369–406.

Anderson, J. R. (1993). Problem solving and learning. *American Psychologist, 48*(1), 35–44.

Baldwin, J. M. (1894). Personality-suggestion. *Psychological Review, 1,* 274–279.

Bartlett, F. C. (1958). *Thinking: An experimental and social study.* New York: Basic Books.

Billett, S. (2001a). Knowing in practice: Re-conceptualising vocational expertise. *Learning and Instruction, 11*(6), 431–452.

Billett, S. (2001b). *Learning in the workplace: Strategies for effective practice.* Sydney, NSW: Allen and Unwin.

Billett, S. (2006). *Work, change and workers.* Dordrecht: Springer.

Billett, S. (2008a). Learning throughout working life: A relational interdependence between social and individual agency. *British Journal of Education Studies, 55*(1), 39–58.

Billett, S. (2008b). Subjectivity, learning and work: Sources and legacies. *Vocations and Learning: Studies in Vocational and Professional Education, 1*(2), 149–171.

Billett, S. (2009). Realising the educational worth of integrating work experiences in higher education. *Studies in Higher Education, 34*(7), 827–843.

Boud, D. , & Solomon, N. (Eds.). (2001). *Work-based learning: A new higher education?.* Buckingham: Open University Press.

Brown, J. S., Collins, A., & Duguid, P. (1989). Situated cognition and the culture of learning. *Educational Researcher, 18*(1), 32–34.

Chi, M. T. H., Feltovich, P. J., & Glaser, R. (1981). Categorisation and representation of physics problems by experts and novices. *Cognitive Science, 5,* 121–152.

Chi, M. T. H., Glaser, R., & Farr, M. J. (1982). *The nature of expertise.* Hillsdale, NJ: Erlbaum.

Department of Innovation Universities and Skills. (2008). *Higher education at work.*

Eames, C., & Coll, R. (2010). Cooperative education: Integrating classroom and workplace learning. In S. Billett (Ed.), *Learning through practice* (pp. 180–196). Dordrecht: Springer.

Engestrom, Y., & Middleton, D. (1996). Introduction: Studying work as mindful practice. In Y. Engestrom, D. Middleton (Eds.), *Cognition and communication at work* (pp. 1–15). Cambridge, UK: Cambridge University Press.

Ericsson, K. A. (2006). The influence of experience and deliberate practice on the development of superior expert performance. In K. A. Ericsson, N. Charness, P. J. Feltowich, & R. R. Hoffmann (Eds.), *The Cambridge handbook of expertise and expert performance* (pp. 685–705). Cambridge: Cambridge University Press.

Ericsson, K. A., & Lehmann, A. C. (1996). Expert and exceptional performance: Evidence of maximal adaptation to task constraints. *Annual Review of Psychology, 47,* 273–305.

Ericsson, K. A., & Smith, J. (1991). *Towards a general theory of expertise.* Cambridge: Cambridge University Press.

Giddens, A. (1991). *Modernity and self-identity: Self and society in the late modern age.* Stanford, CA: Stanford University Press.

Glaser, R. (1984). Education and thinking – The role of knowledge. *American Psychologist, 39*(2), 93–104.

Glaser, R. (1989). Expertise and learning: How do we think about instructional processes now that we have discovered knowledge structures?. In D. Klahr & K. Kotovsky (Eds.), *Complex information processing: The impact of Herbert A. Simon* (pp. 289–317). Hillsdale, NJ: Erlbaum & Associates.

Groen, G. J., & Patel, P. (1988). The relationship between comprehension and reasoning in medical expertise. In M. T. H. Chi, R. Glaser, & R. Farr (Eds.), *The nature of expertise* (pp. 311–342). New York: Erlbaum.

Grollman, P., & Tutschner, R. (2006). *Possible intended and unintended effects of European VET policies – The case of integrating work and learning*. Paper presented at the European Research Network in Vocational Education and Training Symposium, Geneva.

Grubb, W. N., & Badway, N. (1998). *Linking school-based and work-based learning: The implications of LaGuardia's co-op seminars for school-to-work programs*. Berkeley, CA: National Center for Research in Vocational Education.

Larkin, J., McDermott, J., Simon, D. P., & Simon, H. A. (1980). Expert and novice performance in solving physics problems. *Science, 208*(4450), 1335–1342.

Lave, J., Murtaugh, M., & de la Roche, O. (1984). The dialectic of arithmetic in grocery shopping. In B. Rogoff & J. Lave (Eds.), *Everyday cognition: Its development in social context* (pp. 76–94). Cambridge, MA: Harvard University Press.

Lee, Y. J., & Roth, W. -M. (2005). The (unlikely) trajectory of learning in a salmon hatchery. *Journal of Workplace Learning, 17*, 243–254.

Lomas, L. (1997). The decline of liberal education and the emergence of a new model of education and training. *Education + Training, 39*(3), 111–115.

Mezirow, J. (1981). A critical theory of adult learning and education. *Adult Education, 32*(1), 3–24.

Newton, J., Billett, S., Jolly, B., & Ockerby, C. (2009). Journeying through clinical placements – An examination of six student cases. *Nursing Education Today, 29*(6), 630–634.

Perkins, D., Jay, E., & Tishman, S. (1993). Beyond abilities: A dispositional theory of thinking. *Merrill-Palmer Quarterly, 39*(1), 1–21.

Piaget, J. (1968). *Structuralism*. (C. Maschler, Trans. and Ed.). London: Routledge & Kegan Paul.

Rogoff, B. , Lave, J. (Eds.). (1984). *Everyday cognition: Its development in social context*. Cambridge, MA: Harvard University Press.

Ryle, G. (1949). *The concept of mind*. London: Hutchinson University Library.

Schutz, A. (1970). *On phenomenology and social relations (Ed. Helmut Wagner)*. Chicago: University of Chicago Press.

Scribner, S. (1984). Studying working intelligence. In B. Rogoff & J. Lave (Eds.), *Everyday cognition: Its development in social context* (pp. 9–40). Cambridge, MA: Harvard University Press.

Shuell, T. J. (1990). Phases of meaningful learning. *Review of Educational Research, 60*(4), 531–547.

Stenstrom, M.-L., Grollman, P., Tutschner, R., Tynjala, P., Nikkanen, P., & Loogma, K. (2006). *Integration of work and learning: Policies, strategies and practices*. Paper presented at the European Research Network in Vocational Education and Training Symposium, Geneva.

Stevenson, J. (1994). Vocational expertise. In J. Stevenson (Ed.), *Cognition at work* (pp. 7–34). Adelaide, SA: National Centre for Vocational Education Research.

Valsiner, J. (1998). *The guided mind: A sociogenetic approach to personality*. Cambridge, MA: Harvard University Press.

Valsiner, J. (2000). *Culture and human development*. London: Sage.

Valsiner, J., & van der Veer, R. (2000). *The social mind: The construction of an idea*. Cambridge, UK: Cambridge University Press.

Van Lehn, V. (1989). Towards a theory of impasse-driven learning. In H. Mandl & A. Lesgold (Eds.), *Learning issues for intelligent tutoring systems* (pp. 19–41). New York: Springer.

von Glasersfeld, E. (1987). Learning as a constructive activity. In C. Janvier (Ed.), *Problems of representation in the teaching and learning of mathematics* (pp. 3–17). Hillsdale, NJ: Lawrence Erlbaum.

Voss, J. F. (1987). Learning and transfer in subject matter learning: A problem-solving model. *International Journal of Educational Research, 11*(6), 607–622.

Part I
Integrating Practice and University Experiences: Curriculum and Pedagogy Practices

Chapter 3
Preparing Nurses and Engaging Preceptors

Jennifer M. Newton, Stephen Billett, Brian Jolly, and Cherene Ockerby

3.1 Introduction

This chapter examines the preparation of undergraduate student nurses to become functioning registered nurses through their experiences in practice settings. Learning in the health professional setting is such that no two individuals undertaking the same health professional course at the same institution experience or are exposed to identical education and learning (Darcy Associates, 2009). The healthcare workforce is a complex entity that provides ongoing challenges for the preparation of professionals. Nursing comprises the largest component of the Australian health sector's workforce and there are significant problems with preparing, recruiting and retaining nurses (Sheumack, Turner, Brooks, & Moloney, 2008). These problems include the following: (i) existing models of initial nursing education not being wholly effective in developing nursing capacities and identities required for effective nursing work; (ii) nursing work not always providing adequate space for effective professional development; (iii) the formation of a positive professional identity that engages and sustains the working life of nursing not being realised through practice; and (iv) differences in the institutional practices of nurse education institutions and hospitals working against the provision of effective initial and ongoing development of nurses' work. Furthermore, the health sector is faced with shortages partly associated with the high attrition of new graduates (McMeeken, Grant, Webb, Krause, & Garnett, 2008) and the retirement of the 'ageing baby boomer' healthcare workforce within the next decade (Schofield, Page, Lyle, & Walker, 2006). Several authors have proposed that current generational spread across the healthcare workforce is influencing staff development and retention (Boychuk Duchscher & Cowin, 2004; Clausing, Kurtz, Prendeville, & Walt, 2003). Collectively, these problems constitute a complex challenge for those concerned with developing nurses' practice, learning, identity and sustainable institutional practices to ensure that nurses develop and maintain a continuing sense

J.M. Newton (✉)
School of Nursing and Midwifery, Monash University, Melbourne, VIC, Australia
e-mail: jenny.newton@monash.edu

S. Billett, A. Henderson (eds.), *Developing Learning Professionals*, Professional
and Practice-based Learning 7, DOI 10.1007/978-90-481-3937-8_3,
© Springer Science+Business Media B.V. 2011

of worth about their work within the health sector. Hence, it is important to identity practices that can support novice nurses in learning the capacities to become and
identify strongly with being a nurse. This is essential to enable individuals to deliver
quality patient care.

Certainly, the affordances or invitational qualities of support and engagement
offered to student nurses and their capacity to engage with the clinical learning
environment are critical to the quality of students' experience. One tertiary healthcare facility in metropolitan Melbourne, Australia, in partnership with a school
of nursing and midwifery from a major university, sought to augment students'
engagement in learning through enhancing a model of preceptorship (i.e. support
provided by a more experienced nurse) and continuity in student nurse development by providing clinical experiences in the same hospital setting. The concept
of preceptorship is explored in this chapter as a premise to examining workplace
learning for nursing. The worth and qualities of preceptorship are discussed in the
context of a 3-year study that illuminated the distinctive journeys that both novice
and experienced nurses undertook in their preparation to either become a nurse or
engage in being a preceptor. The intricacies of workplace learning in relation to individuals' dispositions, the level of engagement with available learning opportunities
and the receptiveness of the workplace to the novice are discussed here in arguing
for the case of a learning practice supported through a partnership model of learning. Central issues emerging here refer to creating learning opportunities, gaining
independence by the novice, participation as a team member and overcoming the
intergenerational differences that compound the complexities of the nursing workforce. Pedagogical strategies are suggested that will enhance the contributions of
both the academic institution and healthcare organisation in realising the potential
of both novice and practitioner in professional learning.

3.2 Preceptorship

Research on the clinical environment has consistently and long highlighted the
importance of positive clinical experiences to enable effective professional learning to occur (Martin & Happell, 2001; Rushworth & Happell, 2000). Much of the
responsibility for providing positive learning experiences for students in the clinical
setting falls to experienced practitioners who work alongside novice practitioners
or students to facilitate their occupational assimilation into a community of practice
(Wenger, 1998). There are various approaches to providing this support for students.
A common strategy in contemporary nursing is preceptorship (Maclellan & Lordly,
2008). Preceptorship tends to be a short-term workplace relationship between a
novice and an experienced and competent role model focusing on orientation to
the work environment, the teaching of clinical skills, and growth and development of novices' professional capacities (Firtko, Stewart, & Knox, 2005; Kaviani &
Stillwell, 2000). This differs from another commonly used approach of mentorship
which typically involves a long-term relationship focusing on professional development and career progression that extends beyond the clinical setting (Firtko et al.,

2005). The worth of preceptorship as a developmental model resides in the close guidance provided by the more experienced practitioner to the novice. Preceptorship as a model for fostering clinical learning has been widely adopted in Australia, the United Kingdom, and North America. The preceptorship model also aims to increase collaboration between the university that hosts students and the healthcare setting in which they practice by assigning a student to an experienced clinical nurse on a one-to-one basis (Charleston & Happell, 2006; Pickens & Fargotstein, 2006), thereby providing a bridge between two quite distinct settings in which student nurses learn.

The preparation and support of registered (i.e. qualified) nurses to become preceptors is essential in sustaining the provision of effective, high quality learning experiences that meet novices' learning objectives. Formal preparation is often recommended for preceptors so that they are prepared for and become committed to the role of preceptor (Kaviani & Stillwell, 2000; Yonge & Myrick, 2004). This is particularly pertinent given that nurses, like other practice-based professionals, commonly undertake a role in supporting novices in addition to their existing duties and responsibilities (Maclellan & Lordly, 2008; Walker, Cooke, & McAllister, 2008). Assisting in the development of the new entrants is often an expectation of healthcare professionals, as with many others. However, nurses who constantly precept novice nurses are at risk of burnout, unless appropriate support and recognition is provided (Dibert & Goldenberg, 1995; Yonge, Krahn, Trojan, Reid, & Haase, 2002). Feelings of guilt are also reported by preceptors who are torn between providing quality care for their patients and effective learning experiences for novices (Walker et al., 2008; Yonge et al., 2002). This competition between responsibilities can be a source of stress for preceptors (Shannon et al., 2006; Yonge et al., 2002), specifically when dealing with novices who require extensive close supervision and guidance (Dalton, Baker, & Walker, 2004; Gizara & Forrest, 2004; Yonge et al., 2002). Despite these issues, preceptors refer to the rewards and benefits of preceptorship, such as the satisfaction derived from seeing novices' knowledge and skills improve, and the importance of remaining 'up-to-date' with contemporary practice (Shannon et al., 2006). Preceptors also report valuing the opportunity to assist novices' integration into the nursing team and share their own knowledge and skills (Dibert & Goldenberg, 1995).

More than having interest in the role, effective preceptors are those that demonstrate characteristics that include being competent, organised, supportive, motivating, and approachable with strong interpersonal skills (Zilembo & Monterosso, 2008), with the preceptor's leadership style being particularly influential on the quality of novices' experiences and learning (Lockwood-Rayermann, 2003).

An important derivative of preceptorship is learning about professional socialisation. Different definitions of professional socialisation exist, and they consistently emphasise the acquisition of knowledge, skills, values, attitudes and beliefs and commitment to the profession (Maclellan & Lordly, 2008). In essence, professional socialisation is about the learners' acquisition of socially derived knowledge of how one should act in particular practice situations (De Bellis, Longson, Glover, & Hutton, 2001), or what Egan and Jaye (2009), drawing on Wenger's communities

of practice concept, refer to as 'learning professional role boundaries and juris-
dictions' (p. 118). A key component of health professional students' learning is
adapting teachings from the academic setting and making situational adjustments
to the clinical environment. Students' ability to translate the knowledge learned in
the academic setting into practice in the clinical workplace is shaped by personal,
social and environmental factors. These include the students' experiences, interests
and capacities and the invitational qualities of the workplace, plus the particular
practice requirements of that setting. These factors are located in both university
and clinical settings and impact on the richness of the learning experiences and the
potential for translation between these two settings. This translation into practice
can be developed through role modelling and interactions with a range of professionals. The findings from the study of nurses and preceptors identified three factors
that influence this translation of learning through the partnership of a preceptor clinical placement model in nursing. These are creating an environment that supports
learning opportunities; providing learning opportunities and generational tensions.
A consideration of these three factors follows and leads to a model of effective
practice-based learning: strategies for developing a learning partnership.

3.3 Creating an Environment That Supports Learning Opportunities

3.3.1 Learning – A Reciprocal Process

A key basis for affording novice nurses a productive engagement within clinical
settings is creating an environment that is invitational for them to participate in and
learn. This extends to becoming members, albeit peripherally, of the nursing team.
Indeed, becoming part of the nursing team is often a central focus of the novice's
learning as they likely want to be accepted as credible by their co-workers. This
goal, often achieved through the support offered by a more experienced nurse, is
critical to becoming part of that team, which requires them to appropriate the culture and profession of nursing: the culture of practice (Brown, Collins, & Duguid,
1989). Preceptors (i.e. registered nurses) indicate that they derive satisfaction from
welcoming novice nurses to their ward and integrating them into the professional
team. Margaret, an experienced nurse and preceptor, identified that it is not always
necessary to try and teach students: 'oh this drug does that and the side effects
are that ... my role is more, "this is how you be a nurse"'. Students also recognise that the role of the preceptor encompasses more than simply teaching skills
as Jill, a third-year student describes: 'they're the ones that are supposed to help
you integrate into the hospital, so they're like your right hand.' Creating a sense of
belongingness for the novice in the workplace is an important concept that has been
identified as central in promoting clinical learning (Levett-Jones & Lathlean, 2008;
Levett-Jones, Lathlean, Maguire, & McMillan, 2007). As Twentyman, Eaton, and
Henderson (2006) identify, the positive attitudes of individual staff, the ward culture
and the influence of role models are all important in supporting clinical learning.

Preceptors' interest in engaging with novices and actively seeking out learning opportunities is also central to the productive engagement of the novice and is highly valued by the novice. Whilst preceptors might provide diverse learning experiences in the workplace, students recognised that engagement in learning opportunities is a reciprocal process. For example, Stef, a third-year student, valued preceptors who were 'interested in and willing to help you learn', but she also acknowledged that it was vital for her to engage with the opportunities provided: 'I think it's a two way street.'

Some registered nurses also recognised that being a preceptor was a means of enhancing their own clinical knowledge and that they learn alongside their students. For example, Rose, a preceptor, shared: 'sometimes when they [students] ask something or they query something, I have to go and look it up too which I don't mind doing because that also shows up what you know and don't know.'

This willingness to engage in a preceptoring partnership is a critical component of learning in the workplace as Ben, a second-year student, remarked: 'preceptoring is everything . . . a good preceptor can make or break a clinical placement.' Thus, the influence of the experienced professional is pivotal for learning to occur. As Boud, Cohen, & Walker (1993) suggest, 'learning can only occur if the experience of the learner is engaged' (p. 8). In this way, creating an environment in which preceptors are willing to accept novices who in turn believe they are accepted can do much to make the workplace an effective learning environment.

3.3.2 Recognising the Uniqueness of the Individual

As identified above, engagement in learning through preceptorship is premised on a reciprocal process. This process, however, is enhanced for novice nurses if their preceptors relate to them as individuals and recognise their personal knowledge and skill level. In particular, participants in our study identified the importance of preceptors being familiar with a range of learning styles, and recognising novices as unique individuals. A second-year student, Jayne, articulated that it is important that preceptors acknowledge: 'each student as an individual in deciding what they can and can't do, recognising a person as someone unique.' Preceptors who take time to understand the level of support required and familiarise themselves with novices' particular learning style are appreciated by novices. Indeed, our research suggests that preceptors who demonstrated a capacity to understand the particular readiness and learning needs of the student were more likely to be nurses who enjoyed the role of a preceptor. Understanding the variations in individual novices' learning needs can generate more work in supporting and guiding them but, as experienced preceptor Polly suggests, being a preceptor is 'about allowing somebody to to find their own way but guide them safely.'

In guiding novices, many of the preceptors drew upon their personal reflections and recollection of once being a novice themselves in an unfamiliar world of clinical practice. It generated a degree of empathy amongst some preceptors in appreciating the difficulties and dilemmas that novices face in the workplace. This sense of empathy with the novice can assist the preceptor to develop a rapport with their student and enable them to engage effectively with the novice and provide support. This is exemplified by Susan, a preceptor who comments: 'it's very important for them to feel that they're able to come to somebody who they trust and somebody who they can ask those silly questions to without feeling endangered or without feeling silly.' This empathy for novices arose from preceptors' recollections of their own experiences as students, and preceptors' aspirations to provide the kinds of learning opportunities that they themselves valued. Bella, a preceptor, acknowledges: 'I know what bad experiences can be like for them and I think they need staff that are willing to help them and show them the better side of things.'

Thus, getting to know novices as individuals in order to tailor the workplace experiences to novices' learning needs was held as an important aspect of preceptoring by the students and preceptors. Indeed, without an effective preceptor, students can be denied opportunities to practice challenging and complex tasks and instead be restricted to routine tasks in which they already have proficiency (Spouse, 2001). To develop their identity as a nurse and enhance skill acquisition students require well-supported opportunities to extend what they have learnt in university.

3.4 Enhancing Learning Opportunities and Engagement

The importance of the invitational qualities of the workplace in enhancing the translation of learning across the academic and practice setting, to enable novices to develop their knowledge and practical skills, cannot be underestimated. Experienced practitioners need to be aware of providing appropriate and challenging learning opportunities and be flexible in allowing novices to experience different procedures and to practise skills themselves. Third-year student Ellie illustrates this point well: 'If a nurse is sticking in a nasogastric [tube] or if they're taking out the PICC ... think "oh, I've got a student, let's let them do it".' In contrast Eddie, a second-year student, recalled her frustration at not being able to engage: 'some preceptors are very open to you doing it ... Other ones will say come and do this and when you're about to do it they jump in and do it.' This sense of frustration was frequently voiced by student participants in our study, particularly as they neared the completion of their degree and were concerned that the opportunity to practise specific skills or procedures had eluded them. This is illustrated through Ben's experience: 'I haven't got to do an IVC [intravenous cannulation] or a nasogastric [passing a nasogastric tube] ... maybe the next one is yours, regardless of where it was.'

The importance of the nursing staff taking an interest in novices' learning was reported by our participants. In her capacity as a newly registered nurse, Ellie valued: 'having another nurse who's senior to you stop and spend the time to go through things with you properly and comprehensively ... taking time out to supervise you doing a procedure, and then allowing you to become independent at it.' Workplaces that create learning opportunities are likely to be generative of rich learning that promotes the development of a dependent novice to an independent practitioner through the acquisition of knowledge, skills and confidence (Henderson, Winch, & Heel, 2006).

Novices' development of confidence and independent practice can arise from engagement in a range of experiences that are construed as being both positive and negative. Anna, a second-year student, recalled her experiences of learning to give an injection:

> I took with me some of the insights from my previous placement . . . I had a bad experience the first time I ever did it. The second time I went to do it, I don't know whether it was [because] I'd matured in myself in terms of my skill base and confidence . . . I still had an underlying insight it would be a bad experience but I had exactly the opposite so I actually felt that I'd actually grown.

The benefits of having the opportunity to gain independence in clinical practice become more obvious for students as they progress through their degree into a graduate year. When first interviewed, third-year student Toni indicated that she found it: 'satisfying to actually get to the point where . . . you feel confident enough to actually do it.' As a graduate nurse, Toni noted that her role had now changed: 'instead of being the student I'm able to do a lot more, and I'm allowed to do a lot more independently.' This growth in confidence over the trajectory of being a student enables the novice to engage more effectively as a member of the nursing team as they gradually gain acceptance by the team members through the increasing capacity to contribute meaningfully to the work. The student is able to move beyond the nascent position in which they initially find themselves as a peripheral member of a ward team. This gaining of acceptance is illustrated through the following accounts of Ellie, Eddie and Sally.

Despite being an articulate, mature-age student, Ellie was uncomfortable about contributing to team discussions in her capacity as a student. Ellie was very conscious of being a student and only on a clinical placement for 2–3 few weeks as she reported:

> You sit there in handover . . . you really don't say much. You might put one or two comments in, but you're very aware of the fact that you're a transient in there and you don't want to overstep that boundary.

Similarly, despite being an experienced enrolled nurse, Eddie was also intimidated by the nursing staff on her clinical placements. She recalled an occasion when she was at Hospital B: 'I walked into the handover room and sat down and not a word was said to me. It was very hard, coming into an established team and they'll all know each other and have their ways of doing things . . .' She claimed, 'within nursing it can be quite cliquey and if you don't feel part of it, it is hard to be thinking about what you're doing.'

Sally's journey from third-year student through to graduate nurse shows a clear progression towards becoming part of the nursing team. When first interviewed as a second-year student, Sally commented: 'I try to help other members of the team out where I am but I don't really feel quite part of the team yet.' Towards the end of her third year, Sally recalled that she 'felt a lot more part of the team . . . taking on your own patient load really makes you feel as if you know you can do this next year.'

By the time Sally was working as a graduate nurse she stated: 'I probably feel more supported being a graduate now because I think the staff make you feel more part of the team. As a student, you're always a little bit on the outer because you're only there for a certain amount of time.' In this way, becoming a member of the team arises through productive participation.

Becoming part of the team is an important aspect of the novice's learning in the workplace. It can be considered through Eraut's (2004) two perspectives of learning and knowledge: the individual and the social. The individual perspective enables us to explore how people learn and the differences they bring to the interpretation of their learning. The social perspective offers insights to the expanse of cultural practices and products afforded to the individual in the workplace. This cultural knowledge is generally acquired informally through participatory practices which, in the cases of the novices presented here, are seen in part through acceptance as a team member. However, a difficulty realised in the current healthcare workplace that can influence the degree of engagement for both the novice and the experienced practitioner is intergenerational diversity.

3.5 Generational Tensions

Whilst multigenerational diversity is not a new phenomenon it is often exacerbated in current nursing workforces (Clausing et al., 2003). These workforces currently comprise four generations of nurses, each with its distinct perspectives on nursing (Clausing et al., 2003; Martin, 2004). A fifth generation, those born post-1990, will soon also be part of the workforce. Each generation is characterised and shaped by the social, political, and historical events that implicitly shape generational members' underlying core values and work ethic that can influence professional work behaviour (Boychuk Duchscher & Cowin, 2004).

Whilst not all individuals fit the mould for their generational cohort, they generally share some common beliefs, values and attitudes that are shaped by their life experiences (Clausing et al., 2003; Lavoie-Tremblay, O'Brien-Pallas, Gelinas, Desforges, & Marchionni, 2008; Martin, 2004; Swearingen & Liberman, 2004). In a constantly changing nursing workplace characterised by globalisation, increasing technology, competition and unpredictable staffing needs (Martin, 2004), these generational differences can lead to tension and conflict in nursing practice (Boychuk Duchscher & Cowin, 2004; Swearingen & Liberman, 2004). However, in the context of learning nursing this potential for conflict is further exacerbated due to the diversity of generations that many of the student cohorts in undergraduate nursing programmes now represent, and how this range of students engage in learning. The confidence and life experience that comes with returning to study at a mature age can be advantageous in regards to interpersonal interactions. For instance, whilst a 20-year-old student may not feel comfortable making demands of nurses or questioning instructions, Anna, who returned to undergraduate study late in her working life (i.e. mid-1950s) identified: 'I have got, I think, a degree of confidence that I was actually able to say to the preceptor ... "no, don't walk off while I am doing this, could you please stay".'

In contrast, a key challenge for younger nursing students was interacting with older, hospital-trained nurses who have never studied at a tertiary level. This group of nurses sometimes appeared to devalue university education and made comments to Toni such as: 'I don't know how you do university.' As a young graduate, Toni identified that this generation does not 'really understand about the transition' from university to clinical settings. Learning to practice in a clinical ward where the prevailing culture was influenced predominately by older nurses became a challenge for members of the younger generations as they were not 'really interested in the same thing they are'. Yet, for older students it is also a challenge as they learn how to manage the reaction of nursing staff to their maturity. A third-year student, Anna, shared the following story of an encounter with a preceptor:

> It's been the most negative experience I've had and part of that has been [because] I'm a mature age student. The preceptor, who happens to be even older than I am, doesn't think I should be here and she asked the question 'why am I doing this? I should just retire and give the place to somebody else.'

Anna explained that this preceptor: 'trained in a hospital 30 years ago overseas and does not support university training'.

Eddie also reported that being older set her apart from the students who had come straight from high school:

> being a bit older and having a bit of life experience I think helps you to make a decision on what you are doing and why you need to be there ... I notice that a lot with the school friends ... they will be sitting in the lecture drawing something and you feel like going 'you know you don't have to be here, you can leave.

As the above accounts illustrate, each individual student is unique in terms of their personal characteristics and experiences. The lack of open invitations for the next generation of nurses does little to support their development of nursing competence and identity. In particular, the negative values and beliefs held by nurses trained in the hospital system towards contemporary nurse education programmes are indicative of the intergenerational tensions that can permeate the nursing workforce. These experiences are consistent with the accounts in the larger student sample in our project and reflect current issues confronting novice nurses in their clinical learning experiences. Thus, the challenge is to develop a positive learning environment that is invitational to the novice. This is an important aspect for consideration given that the novice nurse expects constant feedback, praise and rewards and to be appreciated for their contribution. A recent study highlighted that a key factor in new nurses' intent to quit was the lack of social support from superiors and colleagues (Lavoie-Tremblay et al., 2008). Undergraduate student nurses may well leave the clinical learning environment questioning their choice of a career in nursing when they are made to feel unwelcome due to the nature of their workplace engagement (Curtis, Bowen, & Reid, 2007). Workplace cliques and affiliations can negatively shape learning experiences through exerting some control over student nurses' ability to engage in rich learning opportunities (Newton, Billett, & Ockerby,

2009). For example, Ben stated instances of nurses' indifference to students: 'well the ward I was just on they [students] just weren't recognised by a lot of the staff, they just seemed to be in the way of all the staff.' It is likely that being a student is difficult enough for these novices, without having to negotiate these cliques and affiliations in unfamiliar clinical environments. However, promotion of engagement in learning in healthcare practice can be achieved through the development of a learning practice that encompasses curriculum practices and pedagogic strategies that support the presence of a professional values and practice (Billett & Newton, 2010).

3.6 Strategies for Developing a Learning Partnership

As proposed in this chapter, learning environments are privileged by the kinds of activities and interactions they afford individuals and the individuals' interest in engaging in these learning opportunities. The dynamics of the workplace experience and how individuals are permitted to participate and engage in activities is a key component of their learning (Billett, 2006). Notwithstanding the organisational and cultural milieu of workplaces, the underlying dispositions and values of both the novice and experienced practitioner also have a central role in how learning will take place and be shaped. For the novice, the perceived relevance of the practice-based curriculum, the pedagogic opportunities and the learning strategies used will influence to a considered extent the way in which they engage in learning.

The preparation prior to undertaking a placement experience can influence the engagement of the novice, particularly if it reduces the time required of the experienced practitioner to familiarise the novice with key elements of the workplace. One pedagogical approach utilised within our research project to assist undergraduate students in orientating them to a new clinical placement environment was the introduction of web-based graphic organisers. Graphic organisers are a type of concept map: 'a visual and graphic display that depicts the relationships between facts, terms or ideas within a learning task' (Hall & Strangman, 2002). The use of organisers has been extensively studied, principally in the field of education (Ausubel, 2000). In appearance, graphic organisers are a cluster map of generic information. Preceptors participating in our project identified a greater need to map the clinical management of common health conditions relevant to specific practice settings to enhance the use of students' clinical time and maximise preceptors' engagement with their students. This strategy to advance students' preparation for learning helped the students to identify knowledge gaps before commencing their clinical placements and generated a sense of feeling better prepared for their placement.

Maximising the learning and engagement that can occur in the workplace for student and practitioner can be promoted through the concept of a 'learning practice'. The premise of this concept is that learning can be conducted in workplaces as part of everyday professional work (Billett & Newton, 2010). Take the example of Eddie who experienced walking into a staffroom for the handover (a nursing practice where one finishing shift of staff gives a verbal report on the patients to the incoming shift staff) and not a word was said to her. Here was a situation that, if managed with a different approach, had the potential to be a learning opportunity. It is these situations that can provide access to authentic learning experiences through direct and indirect guidance that are generative of valuable professional knowledge (Billett & Newton, 2010). What Eddie required in that moment was to be welcomed by a member of staff, introduced to the team and provided with a sense of what was expected of her. The guidance that Eddie needed is exemplified in the contrasting account of Leeny, a second-year undergraduate nursing student, who had just completed her first acute care clinical placement:

> I thought it was fantastic in my ward. We got to interact with occupational therapists, the receptionist, the doctors and the pharmacist. . . . we got to see that multidisciplinary team and be a part of it. As a student that was very encouraging. It really opened my eyes as to how important it is to work as a team.

Having this type of support from a variety of members of the healthcare team in guiding the direction of students' practice through the provision of experiences offers an invaluable learning experience. Guidance by more experienced co-workers can assist in developing the kinds of knowledge and skills required for expert performance. However, it requires a reciprocal process of participation by both the guide and the learner (Billett & Newton, 2010).

Workplace learning support is offered through experienced nurses' identifying and organising ways to assist and monitor students' progression and involving them in workplace activities as they progressively develop the skills required for competent performance and expertise (Billett & Newton, 2010). Workplace learning support can be secured through the effortful and appreciative engagement of the learner with the opportunities that arise and are offered through everyday work practices. This type of support is illustrated through the account of Sally, a third-year undergraduate student, who shared one of the learning sources she was able to draw upon. Her interview extract reveals the importance of the invitational quality of the workplace, as well as her ability to take up of that invitation:

> Sometimes the doctors will let you watch a procedure and will explain things, and even physiotherapists and dieticians . . . they are not the main sources but they do give you extra learning material. I'm always interested in learning a new skill and if the preceptor (the registered nurse) makes me feel happy that I'm there and gets me to do these new skills then it is more motivating too that they want me to be there.

Workplace learning support is also about organising a learning curriculum (i.e. a workplace curriculum) that clearly identifies the sequencing and activities that individuals can progress through in order to refine and develop their competence. It is identifying and ensuring that the most is made of pedagogic opportunities. The shift handover, which for Eddie was such a missed opportunity, has the potential to provide a learning moment for practitioners at different levels of competence through offering particularly helpful insights into nursing practices (Billett & Newton, 2010). Such a learning experience was described by Clare during her first rotation as a new graduate nurse:

> You will go and hand over your patients and the nurse-in-charge ends up telling you more than you tell them. I find that really helpful and they are just continuously giving you education and support as you go along.

The use of specific guided learning strategies has been shown to be easily adopted by those who have enjoyed the benefits of professional training and generated a deep understanding of the concepts and procedures that they use in their practice (Billett, 2001). In particular, the importance of selecting the most appropriate strategy when the novice is reliant upon the more experienced practitioner for assistance in a specific area of practice is highlighted in the study reported here. Two examples of effective guided learning strategies are provided below.

During her third year as an undergraduate student nurse, Clare described how a good preceptor guided her learning in undertaking two new clinical skills:

> When you are doing things like taking blood or doing an ECG, what I find helpful is a good preceptor, when I do the skill for the first time, that I can be shown it and then I do it and that someone [the preceptor] is with me. That makes a big difference.

Guidance focuses on the learners' work activities, and is therefore premised on their taking up of this opportunity. In the above example, the collaborative qualities of learning specific procedures are illustrated through the reciprocal process of modelling and demonstrations followed by approximations of the modelled activity by the learner (Billett & Newton, 2010).

Toni, during her third-year clinical placements as a student, undertook a rotation in the operating theatre. Toni *'wanted to go and see everything being done'* and was fortunate that this placement offered her a very hands-on approach which was enhanced by her enthusiasm:

> I worked with a scrub nurse, an anaesthetic nurse and a recovery nurse and they were all really interesting … and even the doctors and the anaesthetist … Because I seemed so eager about it, they just put me in positions and were like, 'okay you can help me intubate then' and I'm like 'what do I do?' and I just helped them and all that kind of thing. … it was somewhere I had never been before. I kind of just asked lots of questions and they kind of put me in the spot. It got to a point in theatre where the doctors pulled out some of the bowel and said 'I think it is an intussusception this is what it looks like' and he pulled it and I am like 'whoa.'

These examples illustrate how engagement can occur with individuals through guided activities that involve the conscious and effortful participation in professional practice (Billett & Newton, 2010). Developing learning through a partnership in professional practice not only requires preparation before and during the experiences for both the novice and experienced practitioner, but also entails ensuring that learning after placement experience is fully utilised. The importance of this aspect is explored in Chapter 7 where the outcomes of a reflective learning group to assist preparation for practice for undergraduate student nurses are discussed.

3.7 Promoting Professional Learning at Work

Using accounts of students and experienced practitioners, this chapter has presented how engagement in learning can be promoted, organised and guided through everyday practices in healthcare workplaces. Three salient elements are critical to this learning partnership (Fig. 3.1). First, there are the personal practices through which

Fig. 3.1 The Newton model
of learning partnership

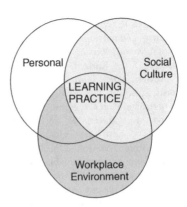

individuals participate and learn. Second, the social culture of the workplace and the tensions that can exist between co-workers can influence the degree of acceptance and subsequent opportunities for learning. Finally, there is the workplace environment, the invitational quality of an individual clinical practice area, the ability to maximise on the informal moments where sharing of knowledge and subsequent learning can take place. Figure 3.1 illustrates the interrelationship between these three elements. If one of these elements generates a degree of disengagement for either the student or practitioner it is likely to create a degree of tension within the workplace that ultimately will influence the potential for learning to occur. As Henderson et al. (2006) acknowledge, professional learning occurs when partnering and learning progress in tandem.

Acknowledgements The author wishes to acknowledge the support provided by the Australian Learning and Teaching Council.

References

Ausubel, D. P. (2000). *The acquisition and retention of knowledge: A cognitive view*. Dordrecht: Kluwer.

Billett, S. (2001). *Learning in the workplace: Strategies for effective practice*. Sydney: Allen and Unwin.

Billett, S. (2006). Constituting the workplace curriculum. *Journal of Curriculum Studies, 38*(1), 31–48.

Billett, S., & Newton, J. M. (2010). Learning practice: Conceptualising professional lifelong learning for the healthcare sector. In N. Frost, M. Zukas, H. Bradbury, & S. Kilminister, (Eds.), *Beyond reflective practice: New approaches to professional lifelong learning* (pp. 52–65). London: Routledge.

Boud, D., Cohen, R., & Walker, D. (1993). *Using experience for learning*. Bristol: The Society for Research into Higher Education and Open University Press.

Boychuk Duchscher, J. E., & Cowin, L. (2004). Multigenerational nurses in the workplace. *Journal of Nursing Administration, 34*(11), 493–501.

Brown, J. S., Collins, A., & Duguid, P. (1989). Situated cognition and the culture of learning. *Education Researcher, 18*(1), 32–42.

Charleston, R., & Happell, B. (2006). Recognising and reconciling differences: Mental health nurses and nursing students' perceptions of the preceptorship relationship. *Australian Journal of Advanced Nursing*, *24*(2), 38–43.

Clausing, S. L., Kurtz, D. L., Prendeville, J., & Walt, J. L. (2003). Generational diversity – the Nexters. *AORN Journal*, *78*(3), 373–379.

Curtis, J., Bowen, I., & Reid, A. (2007). You have no credibility: Nursing students' experiences of horizontal violence. *Nurse Education in Practice*, *7*(3), 156–163.

Dalton, L., Baker, P., & Walker, J. (2004). Rural general practitioner preceptors – how can effective undergraduate teaching be supported or improved? [Electronic Version]. *Rural and Remote Health, 4*. Retrieved July 28, 2008, from http://www.rrh.org.au/publishedarticles/article_print_335.pdf

Darcy Associates. (2009). *Best practice clinical learning environments within health service for undergraduate and early-graduate learners*. Melbourne: Department of Human Services.

De Bellis, A., Longson, D., Glover, P., & Hutton, A. (2001). The enculturation of our nursing graduates. *Contemporary Nurse*, *11*(1), 84–94.

Dibert, C., & Goldenberg, D. (1995). Preceptors' perceptions of benefits, rewards, supports and commitment to the preceptor role. *Journal of Advanced Nursing*, *21*(6), 1144–1151.

Egan, T., & Jaye, C. (2009). Communities of clinical practice: The social organisation of clinical learning. *Health*, *13*(1), 107–125.

Eraut, M. (2004). Informal learning in the workplace. *Studies in Continuing Education*, *26*(2), 247–273.

Firtko, A., Stewart, R., & Knox, N. (2005). Understanding mentoring and preceptorship: Clarifying the quagmire. *Contemporary Nurse*, *19*(1–2), 32–40.

Gizara, S. S., & Forrest, L. (2004). Supervisors' experiences of trainee impairment and incompetence at APA-accredited internship sites. *Professional Psychology – Research and Practice*, *35*(2), 131–140.

Hall, T., & Strangman, N. (2002). Graphic organizers. Retrieved October 25, 2007, from www.cast.org/publications/ncac/ncac_go.html

Henderson, A., Winch, S., & Heel, A. (2006). Partner, learn, progress: A conceptual model for continuous clinical education. *Nurse Education Today*, *26*(2), 104–109.

Kaviani, N., & Stillwell, Y. (2000). An evaluative study of clinical preceptorship. *Nurse Education Today*, *20*(3), 218–226.

Lavoie-Tremblay, M., O'Brien-Pallas, L., Gelinas, C., Desforges, N., & Marchionni, C. (2008). Addressing the turnover issue among new nurses from a generational viewpoint. *Journal of Nursing Management*, *16*(6), 724–733.

Levett-Jones, T., & Lathlean, J. (2008). Belongingness: A prerequisite for nursing students' clinical learning. *Nurse Education in Practice*, *8*(2), 103–111.

Levett-Jones, T., Lathlean, J., Maguire, J., & McMillan, M. (2007). Belongingness: A critique of the concept and implications for nursing education. *Nurse Education Today*, *27*(3), 210–218.

Lockwood-Rayermann, S. (2003). Preceptors, leadership style, and the student practicum experience. *Nurse Educator*, *28*(6), 247–249.

Maclellan, D. L., & Lordly, D. (2008). The socialization of dietetic students: Influence of the preceptor role. *Journal of Allied Health*, *37*(2), 81E–92E.

Martin, C. A. (2004). Bridging the generation gap(s). *Nursing*, *34*(12), 62–63.

Martin, T., & Happell, B. (2001). Undergraduate nursing students' views of mental health nursing in the forensic environment. *Australian and New Zealand Journal of Mental Health Nursing*, *10*(2), 116–125.

McMeeken, J., Grant, R., Webb, G., Krause, K. L., & Garnett, R. (2008). Australian physiotherapy student intake is increasing and attrition remains lower than the university average: A demographic study. *Australian Journal of Physiotherapy*, *54*(1), 65–71.

Newton, J. M., Billett, S., & Ockerby, C. (2009). Journeying through clinical placements: An examination of six student cases. *Nurse Education Today*, *29*, 630–634.

Pickens, J. M., & Fargotstein, B. P. (2006). Preceptorship: A shared journey between practice and education. *Journal of Psychosocial Nursing and Mental Health Services, 44*(2), 31–36.

Rushworth, L., & Happell, B. (2000). 'Psychiatric nursing was great, but I want to be a "real" nurse': Is psychiatric nursing a realistic choice for nursing students?. *Australian and New Zealand Journal of Mental Health Nursing, 9*(3), 128–137.

Schofield, D. J., Page, S. L., Lyle, D. M., & Walker, T. J. (2006). Ageing of the baby boomer generation: How demographic change will impact on city and rural GP and nursing workforce. *Rural and Remote Health, 6*(4), 1–9.

Shannon, S. J., Walker-Jeffreys, M., Newbury, J. W., Cayetano, T., Brown, K., & Petkov, J. (2006). Rural clinician opinion on being a preceptor [Electronic Version]. *Rural and Remote Health, 6*. Retrieved July 28, 2008, from http://www.rrh.org.au/publishedarticles/article_print_490.pdf

Sheumack, M., Turner, C., Brooks, P., & Moloney, B. (2008). *Review of the nursing workforce in Australia* (Vols. 1 and 2). Melbourne: The Australian Health Workforce Institute (AHWI).

Spouse, J. (2001). Bridging theory and practice in the supervisory relationship: A sociocultural perspective. *Journal of Advanced Nursing, 33*(4), 512–522.

Swearingen, S., & Liberman, A. (2004). Nursing generations: An expanded look at the emergence of conflict and its resolution. *Health Care Manager, 23*(1), 54–64.

Twentyman, M., Eaton, E., & Henderson, A. (2006). Enhancing support for nursing students in the clinical setting. *Nursing Times, 102*(14), 35–37.

Walker, R., Cooke, M., & McAllister, M. (2008). The meaningful experiences of being a Registered Nurse (RN) Buddy. *Nurse Education Today, 28*(6), 760–767.

Wenger, E. (1998). *Communities of practice: Learning, meaning, and identity.* Cambridge: Cambridge University Press.

Yonge, O., Krahn, H., Trojan, L., Reid, D., & Haase, M. (2002). Being a preceptor is stressful!. *Journal for Nurses in Staff Development, 18*(1), 22–27.

Yonge, O., & Myrick, F. (2004). Preceptorship and the preparatory process for undergraduate nursing students and their preceptors. *Journal for Nurses in Staff Development, 20*(6), 294–297.

Zilembo, M., & Monterosso, L. (2008). Nursing students' perceptions of desirable leadership qualities in nurse preceptors: A descriptive survey. *Contemporary Nurse, 27*(2), 194–206.

Chapter 4
Targeted Preparation for Clinical Practice

Elizabeth Molloy and Jenny Keating

The key messages I'm getting from this [transition] week are to be proactive in my learning during clinicals in terms of critically reflecting and not leaving it to the supervisor to make times with me for feedback. To be professional and show interest in what I am doing, be punctual and be prepared with notes. To concentrate on the patient rather than the fact that I am being tested and to understand that I am not the priority- the patient is. To be socially aware of people, adapting to my supervisor's style of teaching. (Student 10)

4.1 Introduction

This chapter discusses the efficacy of a week-long curricular initiative, designed to prepare physiotherapy students for their transition to clinical practice. The physiotherapy programme at Monash University is a 4-year degree. The first 2.5 years of this degree programme are based in the University setting and the final 1.5 years are dedicated to learning in practice settings, with students undertaking a total of 42 weeks of practical education. The chapter discusses the implementation and assessment of an innovative 1-week transition programme designed to prepare students for the demands of clinical education. The aims of the transition programme include: (i) to make transparent the expectations of clinical education and (ii) to provide students with further knowledge and skills in self-directed learning as a means of negotiating the complexity and uncertainty of the clinical environment.

Although the transition programme received high satisfaction ratings from students, focus groups involving students held after the completion of the transition week revealed a lack of alignment between educator and student perceptions of transition week activities and objectives that would best prepare students for workplace learning. Educators designed the transition programme with the aim of encouraging learning agency through the development of skills in communication, leadership, and critical thinking. The quote presented above demonstrates that some students

E. Molloy (✉)
Monash University, Melbourne, VIC, Australia
e-mail: Elizabeth.Molloy@monash.edu

S. Billett, A. Henderson (eds.), *Developing Learning Professionals*, Professional and Practice-based Learning 7, DOI 10.1007/978-90-481-3937-8_4,
© Springer Science+Business Media B.V. 2011

recognised these as the target objectives. However, the bulk of the data suggested that students' priorities leading into their first clinical placement reflected a 'survival focus', and a preoccupation with the attainment and demonstration of technical/procedural skills. Survey results supported that students, throughout university-based learning, valued discipline-specific practical classes above case-based learning tutorials, and above nontechnical skill-focused educational initiatives, such as interprofessional learning seminars.

The results of this study suggest that in order to align student and educator agendas, teaching and learning activities designed to promote nontechnical skill development should be contextualised within a clinical focus. Nontechnical skill development should be embedded in clinically relevant activities where students perceive that they are attaining tangible skills with utility and transferability. Physiotherapy students praised learning activities characterised by perceived relevance and authenticity, and examples of such curriculum initiatives designed to engage students are presented in this chapter. An important question arising from this data is 'can we convince students of the value of metacognitive skills as a way to maximise their learning in the workplace?' This chapter serves to untangle the multiple influences on preparation of students for clinical practice, and proposes both a philosophical and pedagogical approach to soften transition to workplace learning.

4.2 Background

The transition programme constitutes a 4-day research-informed curriculum, designed to prepare students to meet the demands of clinical education. The ingredients of this programme, including the objectives, content, and teaching and learning methods grew from a study of existing literature on transition programmes in health professional education (Chumley Olney, Usatine, & Dobbie, 2005; Prince, Boshuizen, van der Vleuren, & Scherpbier, 2005), research on students' experience of physiotherapy clinical education (Molloy, & Clarke 2005; Delany & Molloy, 2009), and informal feedback and formal feedback (Denniston, Molloy, & Nickson, 2010 manuscript submitted for publication) from clinical educators affiliated with the programme. Clinicians' feedback focused on incoming students' readiness for engagement in professional learning, including perceived strengths and gaps in knowledge and skills (Denniston et al., 2010 manuscript in review). Focus group data suggested that clinical educators affiliated with the programme were generally pleased with incoming students' professionalism and enthusiasm for learning, and identified that the biggest gaps in performance related to clinical reasoning, linking treatment to prioritised patient problems, an adequate repertoire of treatment techniques, and skills in note writing. The identified gap in clinical reasoning ability is consistent with studies of transition in medical education where both students and clinical educators have identified deficiencies in clinical reasoning within the authentic practice context (Gordon et al., 2000; Prince, Van De Wiel, Scherpbier, van Der Vleuten, & Boshuizen, 2000; Van Gessel, Nendaz, Vermeulen,

Junod, & Vu, 2003; Windish, 2000). For this reason, a workshop on processes of clinical reasoning, and potential biases in reasoning, was included in the transition programme.

Delany and Molloy's (2009) study on 'what matters to physiotherapy students in clinical education' involved analysis of year 3 student reflective essays on critical incidents in clinical education. Students were asked to choose any incident, or series of events that contributed to their learning in their first year of clinical education (15 weeks of rotations). Of the essays that were analysed ($n = 53$), 28% were related to the theme of death and dying, 23% of essays were written about professional relationships (namely student-supervisor relationships), and 9% were on encounters relating to feedback on student performance. Given that students had freedom to select a topic, the considerable focus on (and articulated anxiety about) relationships in the clinical setting provided further motivation to incorporate explicit analysis and discussion of expectations of clinical learning into the transition curriculum. The number of essays describing inadequacy, and lack of preparation for interactions with critically ill and dying patients, prompted the inclusion of a simulated scenario in the transition week. One of the four scenarios was based on the dying patient, where students were asked to assess and treat the patient, and communicate with the patient's family. The simulated scenario was capped with a reflective debriefing session to discuss reactions and strategies employed.

As part of the reflective essay task, students were asked to write tips for future students who were about to transition to the clinical learning environment (Delany & Molloy, 2009). These tips were incorporated into a session in the transition programme called the 'role of students in clinical education'. The motivation for this inclusion was that student-generated suggestions for transition would carry more weight than tips from educators. In alignment with the ideology that 'hints are more meaningful coming from past students', two members of the 4th-year physiotherapy cohort were asked to sit on a panel to discuss the highlights and pitfalls in workplace learning and potential strategies for maximising clinical learning. The benefit of student-derived advice on transition was reported by Small et al. (2008, p. 7) in a study of medical transition: 'Some of our students commented that it would help to include 4th-year students as co-facilitators in the preclinical training courses to provide their insights based on firsthand experiences into the roles and expectations of students on the team.' The most commonly presented 'survival tips' from the 53 students are summarised in Box 4.1.

Box 4.1 Year 3 students' tips for transition to clinical education

- 'Play the game' (pick up on the expectations of clinical educator and the workplace)
- Be prepared for hard work

- Seek and use feedback during clinical education
- Be assertive in patient interviews
- Time management is vital – plan your day
- Know the multidisciplinary team members
- Be you, and use your knowledge (try not to get overwhelmed with the assessment and supervision process)
- Ask questions

In the transition programme, students were prompted to comment on these 'survival tips' provided by older physiotherapy students. The recommendation that attracted most debate and conjecture by the 3rd-year cohort included the advice on 'playing the game' in clinical education. Some students commented that they had no interest in playing the game, and 'slotting in with their supervisors'. Rather, they stated that they were heading out to clinics in order to learn and apply their theoretical knowledge into practice. Others added to this line of argument and recalled stories of past 3rd-year students bringing cakes for their supervisors, and making sure they turned away from their supervisor if they were anticipating the arrival of a yawn. These comments invited a healthy and ethically fuelled debate within the classroom about what constitutes respect for an educator, the extent to which a learner should be expected to acquiesce to the educator's viewpoint and practice philosophy, and the merits and pitfalls of trying to 'blend into' an established workplace culture. The amount of discussion and interest generated from the one data point presented was in fact a live example of reflective practice in action, and demonstrates that undergraduate students have the capacity, and are willing, to anticipate the complexity of professional practice.

4.3 Lost in Transition

Undergraduate health professional students consistently report feeling underprepared for the complexity and uncertainty of clinical practice (Ansari, 2003; Cupit, 1988; Le Maistre & Pare, 2004; Molloy & Clarke, 2005; Moss & McManus, 1992; Neville & French, 1991). Healthcare work is inexact and unpredictable. Students entering the arena of clinical practice are expected to apply the concepts and procedures they have learnt in university settings to activities in healthcare practice settings, ensure patient safety, and form professional and productive relationships with patients, caregivers, and colleagues. Additionally, as discussed in the section above, students must also navigate overt and covert institutional norms (i.e. both university- and hospital-based practices). Students are required to interpret and respond to the changing expectations and knowledge base of the profession and the wider healthcare community (Delany & Molloy, 2009). Not only do learners need to comprehend and engage with these professional expectations, they are assessed on their achievement of these goals through their performance in practice-based activities that are still quite novel to them. Continuous longitudinal monitoring, feedback, and assessment of physiotherapy students are needed to protect professional standards and to exercise duty of care to patients. Although assessment can drive learning, for some students, close and near continuous surveillance can cause anxiety when coupled with striving for high performance standards (Keating, Dalton, & Davidson, 2009).

Indeed, healthcare students' anxiety about practice experiences is well acknowledged. Studies by Radcliffe and Lester (2003), Prince et al. (2005), and Small et al. (2008) all highlight medical students' reported anxiety in moving from the preclinical to the clinical environment. The reported stress was attributed to stark differences in learning environments (i.e. safe, student-centred versus complex and patient-centred), workload, performance expectations, and changes in teaching styles. Medical students in these three studies all reported feeling underprepared for this transition. In the study by Small et al. (2008) two cohorts of students completed questionnaires on transition; one group completed this questionnaire prior to transition and the other after 9 months of immersion in clinical education. Both groups expressed similar anxieties about their abilities in clinical reasoning and history-taking/physical examination. Interestingly, the older, immersed cohort identified time management and self-care as factors that caused considerable anxiety. Based on Small et al.'s work, we planned and enacted clinical reasoning exercises and sessions addressing student self-care and well-being as part of the transition programme.

Both students and educators have identified 'the hidden curriculum' in clinical education, defined as the implicit expectations and practices of the profession (Henderson, Ferguson Smith, & Johnson, 2005; Rose & Best, 2005; Small et al., 2008). In learning within practice settings, students begin the process of appropriating professional values including the knowledge, skills, and behaviours that are deemed important by the profession (Lave & Wenger, 1991). In the transition programme, older students, clinical educators, and university-based educators were invited to share with students the expectations, nuances, and common pitfalls of novice practice in the workplace. In explicating these handy hints, and/or heuristics, it is hoped that students can become active agents in the education process rather than being subject to a serendipitous and idiosyncratic enculturation into the profession. We hoped to avoid the distraction from learning that occurs when students (through trial and error) gradually deduce performance targets that are expected, but not explicitly stated. We anticipated that by making clear social and educational expectations the level of student anxiety and energy expenditure would be reduced. This initiative in turn would be likely to free up cognitive processes required for knowledge/skill acquisition, generation, and application.

Contemporary education literature advocates the importance of producing self-directed and reflective learners (Higgs, Richardon, & Abrandt Dahlgren, 2004; Kilminster & Jolly, 2000). Although there is a documented consensus that generating students' capacity for self-regulation is a key curricular goal, there is little information, or evidence, to guide methods of achieving this goal (Baxter & Gray, 2001). The literature emphasises *purpose* (e.g. to produce self-directed learners) and not *process* (e.g. how to produce self-directed and self-regulated learners). This transition initiative is driven by the assumption that these self-directed learning skills need to be scaffolded by educators in the academic setting. Ironically, we are arguing for a directed and (in part) didactic mode of teaching of self-directed learning. Facilitating students' development of skills in critical thinking, self-evaluation, and self-regulation, within a safe, academic environment, may aid students' transition into clinical practice, and equip them with the capacity to act as lifelong learners. As Henderson et al. (2005, p. 6) propose, skills such as giving and receiving feedback should be taught both conceptually and practically in the academic curriculum so that 'the use of these skills becomes second nature and not an act of bravery in the clinical setting'. This sentiment that students should be prepared to exercise habit, rather than bravery, in professional learning is a key conceptual driver in this chapter.

The transition programme was enacted as a 1-week university-based preparatory programme undertaken by 3rd-year physiotherapy students prior to entering clinical placements. The transition week was founded on two key objectives: (1) to make transparent the often-implicit expectations of clinical education and (2) to provide students with knowledge and skills in self-directed learning and critical reflection. These skills are likely to empower students in professional learning and to soften the sharp-edged transition between the academic and clinical learning environments. It is anticipated that identifying likely stressors in the clinical learning environment, and collectively devising and rehearsing strategies to meet such demands, will help free cognitive capacity for workplace learning (Molloy 2009).

4.3.1 What Was Enacted

The transition week included teaching and learning around themes that are presented in Table 4.1. These themes incorporate professional processes, roles, and tasks and were explored using different modes of teaching and learning, as indicated in the right column of this table. Of note is that only two of the nine sessions constituted didactic, lecture-style formats, reflecting the 'active learning' philosophy of the transition curriculum.

As was described in the 'background' section of this chapter, empirical research underpinned the development of the transition curriculum, detailed in Table 4.1. Data derived from students' reflective essays and unit evaluation forms, combined with clinical educator responses to the previous cohort of year 3 students, were strong drivers of the curriculum content. For those in the process of developing a tailored transition programme for health professional students, we would encourage this engagement of stakeholders in helping to establish key learning objectives, learning content, teaching and learning methods, and, if relevant, assessment procedures that reflect the curricular aims. In addition to collecting data on educators' and students' experience of clinical education, we consulted the literature on transition programmes to help shape the final package.

Table 4.2 provides an example of the learning objectives for each session in the transition programme.

Table 4.1 Illustrating learning topic and mode of delivery

Learning theme	Mode of teaching and learning
The health system and patient discharge options	Lecture
The clinical educator's role	Panel discussion, workshop, case-based learning
The student's role	Panel discussion, case-based learning
Adult learning and learning preferences	Interactive seminar, case-based learning
Critical reflection	Lecture
Clinical reasoning	Interactive seminar, case-based learning
Feedback and assessment	Workshop, case-based learning
Leadership in clinical practice	Interactive seminar
Technical and nontechnical skill application	Simulated patient scenarios, practical/laboratory sessions

Table 4.2 Examples of learning objectives for transition sessions

Session/lecture	Learning objectives
Lecture: The healthcare system	Appreciate the complexity of services within Victoria's healthcare system
	Describe the funding arrangements and divisions between governments, patients, private institutions, and health insurance schemes
	Understand the role of health economists in the division of funding and resources
	Recognise the purpose and utilisation of workplace statistics by healthcare management
	Discuss the opportunity and pressures to introducing a new programme/class within a physiotherapy unit
	Identify the key policy differences between Australia's federal and alternative governments, and the impact of these changes upon physiotherapy services
Workshop: The clinical educator's role in clinical education	Define the role and responsibilities of the clinical educator in the clinical setting
	Describe the role and responsibilities of the student in the clinical setting
	Recognise the multiple, and, at times, conflicting roles of clinical educators in relation to their clinical, educational, and managerial responsibilities
	Define an effective clinical educator – student relationship including strategies to optimise student learning
	Recognise situations where conflict may arise in the student – clinical educator partnership
	Identify and discuss strategies to optimise student and clinical educator enjoyment and engagement in the clinical education programme

These learning objectives were provided to the session lecturer/facilitator and drove the content covered. As standard practice in the physiotherapy programme at Monash University, the educator presents the learning objectives to learners at the start of the session, and again at the completion of the session, where students can calibrate the degree to which the session objectives have been met either inwardly, or explicitly. This transparency in presenting learning objectives, and asking students to rate the quality of the learning session in meeting these goals, provides students with agency, and encourages students to critically reflect, a key overarching objective of the transition programme. In addition, such transparency of student reflection provides the lecturer/facilitator with direct feedback on the effectiveness of the session.

4.4 Research Methods

4.4.1 Research Design

The informants in this account of the efficacy of the transition programme were year 3 physiotherapy students ($n = 60$) at Monash University. They were surveyed prior to participating in the week-long transition programme. Immediately following the programme they were surveyed again and then again after 15 weeks of their block of clinical education (see Fig. 4.1 below).

This clinical education block was comprised of 5 weeks in each of three core areas of physiotherapy practice (musculoskeletal physiotherapy, cardiorespiratory physiotherapy, and neurological physiotherapy). The electronic survey was anonymous, and sought learners' opinions about their readiness to practice in clinical education, the educational activities that they perceived as most useful in their learning to date, and specifically their expectations (and/or experience) of the transition programme. In designing the evaluation, we thought it was important to capture participants' immediate experience of the transition programme, in addition to gaining

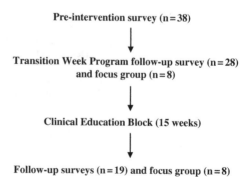

Fig. 4.1 Research design

their opinion on the perceived efficacy of the transition programme after their time immersed in clinical practice.

In addition to the three surveys, a focus group was held with eight students immediately after the transition programme and after the 15 weeks of clinical practice, as a way of capturing rich data on learners' reactions to and experiences of the transition programme. Such in-depth responses could not be elicited from a written survey alone. In focus group one, participants were asked to articulate their expectations of clinical education (see Box 4.2 below), and in the final focus group, the participants were asked about the match between their expectations and their experience of clinical placements.

Box 4.2 Focus group one questions (immediately following the transition programme)

Preparing physiotherapy students for clinical practice: evaluating the 'transition programme' model.

- Welcome and introductions
- What are your expectations re clinical placements? What do you see as your role in clinical placements?
- To what extent do you feel ready to meet the demands and requirements of clinical education?
- What potential difficulties or tensions might you encounter in the clinical learning environment?
- To date in the physiotherapy programme, what learning activities do you see as best helping you to prepare for clinical practice? (May require prompting, e.g. CBL, brief clinical observations, lectures, etc.)
- What did you anticipate to be the purpose of the transition programme?
- To what extent did you feel that the transition programme met these aims?
- What did you find most valuable during the week-long programme? Why?
- What did you find least valuable during the programme? Why?
- What recommendations would you suggest to improve the quality of learning resulting from this transition programme?
- Summarise and conclude session.

The second focus group followed a similar line of questioning, although the focus shifted from capturing the students in an anticipatory mode, to capturing their actual experience of clinical education, and perceived preparation for meeting these challenges.

4.4.1.1 Outcome Measures

Perceived Readiness for Practice

Students were asked to complete a survey and rate their perceived level of readiness for practice before and after the transition programme intervention.

Value of the Transition Programme

Students were asked to appraise the value of the 1-week transition programme in preparing them for the clinical environment both immediately following the intervention, and after 15 weeks of clinical education. Students were provided with opportunities to suggest changes to the transition programme to better facilitate their transition from the academic to the clinical setting. Both the immediate perceptions of the transition programme were captured along with the retrospective value of the transition programme, given that students were able to draw on 'the realities' of 15 weeks of clinical practice to inform their appraisal.

4.4.1.2 Data Analysis

Quantitative survey data were analysed using descriptive statistics. Focus group and open-ended questionnaire responses were analysed by the first author for themes using a grounded-theory approach (Strauss & Corbin, 1998). The audio-recorded focus group data was transcribed verbatim. The basis of this analysis was 'open coding' and 'axial coding' of data, which are terms given to the interpretative categorisation of data. The transcripts were read, and the codes were collapsed into key themes. Quotations and sections of text were extracted into separate word documents under thematic headings, with the transcript and page number recorded to ensure a reference point was provided. To optimise rigour of analysis, an additional two researchers (second author plus research fellow/project coordinator) reviewed and coded the data, and clarified properties and dimensions of emergent themes. An audit trail was made via documentation of decisions made during data analysis.

4.5 Results and Discussion

This section reports and discusses the findings from the surveys. Table 4.3 below presents students' reactions to the transition programme, and also the students' self-reported readiness for practice at three different intervals – preintervention, postintervention, and post-clinical education.

Table 4.3 shows that 78.8% of students in the sample reported that they 'agreed' and 10.7% 'strongly agreed' that the learning objectives in the transition sessions were achieved. These figures were seen as encouraging, as anecdotal and research-based reports (Chumley et al., 2005; Prince et al., 2005) point to the difficulty in engaging health professional students in learning content that is seen as removed

Table 4.3 Learners' reported experience of transition programme and readiness for practice

	Strongly disagree (%)	Disagree (%)	Neutral (%)	Agree (%)	Strongly agree (%)
The learning objectives in the lectures/workshops were achieved ($n = 28$)	0	0	10.7	78.8	10.7
I feel adequately prepared for clinical education Preintervention ($n = 38$)	0	11.1	42.2	41.7	0
Postintervention ($n = 28$)	0	0	39.3	57.1	3.6
After 15 weeks of clinical education ($n = 19$)	0%	15.8%	42.1%	42.1%	0%

from pure biomedical knowledge/practice. The data in Tables 4.4 and 4.5, however, still indicate that students tend to privilege acquisition of practical skills and biomedical knowledge over learning of professional, communication, and educational skills. The qualitative data collected via focus groups also supports this trend in student engagement and satisfaction with 'the hard sciences' within the university-based curriculum. This concept of engagement in what is perceived as 'peripheral' curricular content is discussed further in this chapter.

Also, indicated in Table 4.3 is students' perceived readiness for practice. Students were asked if they felt adequately prepared for clinical education before the intervention (11% disagree), after the intervention (0% disagree), and, again, after 15 weeks of clinical education (16% disagree). The elevated percentage of students who reported feeling underprepared for practice after the clinical education block

Table 4.4 Learners' ratings of individual transition programme sessions

Topic/activity	Average rating ($n = 28$)
The clinical educator's role	2.36
The student's role	2.39
Practical sessions (technical skill development)	2.46
Clinical reasoning	2.64
Feedback and assessment	2.86
Critical reflection	3.71
Leadership in clinical practice	3.93
The health system and discharge options	4.07
Adult learning and learning styles	4.32

Postintervention survey ($n = 28$) (1 = most helpful, 10 = least helpful).

Table 4.5 Learner ratings of learning activities in university (years 1–3) that have best prepared them for clinical practice (1 = most helpful, 10 = least helpful)

Learning activity	Average rating ($n = 38$)
Practical classes (technical skills)	2.16
CBL	3.08
Lectures	3.16
Private study	3.38
Tutorials	3.69
Written exams	3.95
Assignments	5.32
IPE seminars	6.25

was anticipated. The rationale is that students often report that the shift into clinical practice is more difficult than they had initially anticipated (Cupit, 1988). This mismatch between expectations and experience can be partly explained by the enhanced understanding of scope of practice that occurs through immersion in practice itself. That is, prior to clinical education, students' conception of the target (i.e. what it means to perform as a competent physiotherapist) is largely an academic conception, rather than a construction based on observation of expert practice or immersion in practice.

Table 4.4 displays the learners' ratings (perceived utility) of each of the sessions in the transition programme, where 1 = most helpful and 10 = least helpful. All of the sessions were rated on the 'helpful' side of the spectrum, with learning about the clinical educator's role and the student's role viewed as the most helpful.

The other learning activity that was rated particularly highly by students in the transition programme was the practical skills sessions that focused on technical skill acquisition (Table 4.4). These practical sessions included physical assessment and management techniques for common conditions across cardiothoracic, musculoskeletal, and neurological practice domains. The data presented in Table 4.5 below reflect a similar pattern of the relative privileging of practical classes in the curriculum. In this particular question on the survey, students were asked to rate learning activities throughout the 3 years of the course that best contributed to their preparation for practice. 'Hands on' practical classes were rated above learning modes such as case-based learning tutorials and lectures as contributing most to their learning and readiness for professional practice.

The survey results broadly supported the proposition that students, throughout their 2.5 years of university-based learning, valued discipline-specific practical classes above nontechnical skill-focused educational initiatives, such as interprofessional learning seminars, that are designed to promote skills in teamwork, leadership, and communication. This tendency for learners to privilege technical or procedural skill acquisition over development of 'nontechnical' knowledge or skill (e.g. communication, ethics, reflective practice, adult learning) also emerged as a strong theme in the focus group data discussed below.

4.5.1 Themes from Qualitative Data Analysis

In the following section, the findings and deductions arising from data that focused on the key themes are described and discussed with reference to literature on health professional education.

4.5.1.1 Theme 1: Differences in Intended, Enacted, and Experienced Curriculum

Student Diagnosis of 'Peripheral' Curricular Content

There is a discourse in the education literature devoted to the gap between the intended, enacted, and experienced curriculum (Billett, 2006). There can be a dissonance between the overarching aims of teaching and learning, the way in which educators operationalise the curriculum, and the way that learners themselves *experience* the curriculum. The Monash physiotherapy programme is explicit in five themes or threads that contribute to the professional practice skill set (see Table 4.6). These themes are vertically integrated across the 4-year programme and horizontally integrated around weekly cases in preclinical semesters. The five threads of knowledge are used to balance curriculum content and provide learners with a clear map of the domains of knowledge that are considered important for clinical practice.

Despite explicitly targeting the five themes with learning tasks, and integrating skills across themes in weekly curriculum design, learners do not appear to engage with all curricular elements with equal endeavour or enthusiasm. Health professional educationalists writing about 'reflective practice' often point to their 'uphill battle' in convincing undergraduate students of the importance of reflective skills as an integral, rather than peripheral, part of practice (Delany & Molloy, 2009; Driessen, van Tartwijk, Overeem, Vermunt, & van der Vleuten, 2005).

> We argue that for students to develop habits of critical reflection in their professional practice, they must be exposed to explicit teaching of reflective practice principles, along with modeling of critical reflection by university and clinically-based educators .... By making transparent to students the transformative nature of reflective practice, through listening to students' recommendations and acting on these recommendations, reflection is conceptualised as a key *part of practice* rather than positioned as a retrospective metacognitive activity. (Delany & Molloy, 2009, p. 26)

Table 4.6 Themes in the Monash physiotherapy curriculum

Theme number	Description
Theme 1	Personal and professional practice
Theme 2	Population, society and health
Theme 3	Fundamental knowledge of health science
Theme 4	Applied practice
Theme 5	Research

Delany and Molloy (2009) argue that students' lack of engagement in educational activities aimed at developing reflective practice can be attributed to poor curricular design, and inadequate modelling by educators. If reflection is introduced late in the programme, and is positioned as a skill removed from clinical decision-making and clinical practice, then it will indeed be treated as a skill peripheral to 'core business'. In many health professional programmes, reflective practice is developed via once-off reflective essays, with little instruction or theoretical framework underpinning the task. Often reflective tasks are not formally assessed, which can again reinforce to students the sentiment that reflective skills are external to core practice competencies. In addition, the transformative nature of reflection is often hidden to students. For example, if students rate a unit poorly, educators make corresponding changes to the teaching materials or approach, based on the feedback. By making transparent to the students the resultant changes to the curriculum, educators are modelling reflective practice, and positioning students as agents of change in the process.

The findings from this transition programme research illustrate the gaps between curricular intentions and students' experience. In the transcript below, students label knowledge framed under 'Personal and professional development' (theme one) as peripheral or 'iffy'. There is no need to reverse engineer the concept of 'iffy' and to hypothesise what students define as the knowledge central to their attainment of practice competence. In the data, students defined this with swift confidence, without prompting. Both the survey data and focus group data point to 'non-iffy' learning as development of technical or procedural skills such as a knee joint physical assessment or neurological testing of sensation, muscle power, and reflexes. Table 4.6 reveals that students identified practical classes as the most helpful method of learning in their university-based section of the degree programme.

The following passage from the focus group data reflects students' evaluation of the transition week, and includes viewpoints on what they see as peripheral, or 'nonessential' elements of the physiotherapy curriculum.

Facilitator: What do you see as the purpose of preclinical week?
Male: Gets us ready for clinics.
Female: Getting ready for clinics.
Female: Preparation.
Male: Covering all those little things that we never thought about, like . . .
Female: The stuff that's not really linked to physio that's more linked to us professionally or how we behave or. . .
Female: Yeah, that kind of like feedback and evaluating.
Male: And linking everything all together.
Facilitator: Mmmm
Male: Our professionalism and our knowledge and our . . . .
Facilitator: Yes. So what do you mean by professionalism?
Male: How to act toward the patient, towards the clinical staff, looking from their side
Female: Not just the patients, you know, the family . . . .
Female: The patient's family, I never thought of that.
Facilitator: So, had you thought of these issues before or did you feel like they're new?
Male: No.
Male: Not really.

Male:	Even the feedback session, like I never imagined there'd be so much complexity, I thought it would be just like, yeah feedback, but just be introduced to this whole like array of things that can be problematic about it, that it's just something that you would have just taken for granted if I hadn't come to this week.
Facilitator:	Hmm. So, if we say that's the purpose, and to what extent do you think that purpose has been met by this week?
Male:	Awareness has definitely been developed or at least introduced, like as I said, I wouldn't even have thought of half the things.
Female:	Yep.
Male:	Given us the basic concepts and depending on our own thoughts we'll, in our own clinical experiences later on, will develop them.
Facilitator:	Hmm. Because a lot of the content has been around professionalism, adult learning, so, as you said those 'nonclinical' if you like, themes, did you feel frustrated at any point, or did you struggle to see the relevance?
Male:	I found the lectures sort of iffy.
Male:	Like because I know that we had a lot of stuff on ethics and the legal system and stuff in first year and no one pays attention because they can't see . . .
Female:	The relevance.
Male:	There's no sort of application of the legal and ethical implications, like she tried to make practical examples but . . .
Female:	Like they tell us about these issues but they don't actually do the application side of it.
Female:	Those iffy topics, they were ok but again, like they'd even be more useful when you're out in the clinics because I know that the group that I was in . . . they were like 'why are we doing this, this is stupid, rah rah rah, this is a waste of my time.'
Facilitator:	Mmm. So does it help you if your lecturer or your tutor can say this is why this is important? Does that, is that a key?
Female:	Very key.

During this discussion, students identified the likely value of this 'iffy' material, and hypothesised that they would recognise the relevance of such knowledge once they embarked on clinical rotations. Some participants acknowledged the importance of educators sign posting important material, for example 'you need to know this material in order to . . . .'. The student data prompts further discussion about when is the right time to introduce theme-one concepts to students. That is, would students benefit from earlier exposure to the clinical practice environment to better understand the relevance of these communication- or professionalism-based skills? Or do educators need to exercise more craft in embedding theme-one learning objectives within clinically based scenarios, so that students see these areas as core business in physiotherapy? Or should students be introduced to ethical issues much later in the curriculum when there is a clear application for the knowledge? There needs to be more dialogue and more research surrounding the timing and methods in teaching these skills in health professional programmes.

The students were asked for their suggestions to improve the transition programme, both immediately after the intervention, and after 15 weeks of clinical immersion. The recommendations fell neatly into two categories: (i) more practical sessions, and therefore more opportunities to develop technical/procedural skills, and (ii) less lecture material and more interaction. In doing so, students pointed to the tensions between didactic teaching of foundational/canonical knowledge and application of knowledge (interactive learning). The transition programme was founded on sequencing of learning, whereby students were exposed to theoretical principles (e.g. models of feedback) and were then provided with opportunities for applying these principles (e.g. providing feedback to their peer in an interactive role play). While learners may not provide overwhelmingly flattering *feedback* on the provision of 'fundamental principles' as a platform for learning, the question remains as to whether learners first need exposure to concepts before application of concepts. Our stance is that there may be merit in holding a 'middle ground' position whereby factual material is interwoven with interactive modes of learning. This middle way is reflected in the majority of health professional programmes whereby problem-based learning is enacted in a hybrid form, alongside the provision of related didactic lectures (Davis & Harden, 1999).

Demonstrating the power of hindsight, students reported that they did not see the relevance of learning certain aspects of conceptual material until they had engaged in clinical practice. Such reflections reinforce the importance of an integrated teaching approach where 'nontechnical' skill development should be embedded in clinically relevant activities where students perceive that they are attaining tangible skills with utility and transferability. Physiotherapy students praised learning activities characterised by perceived relevance and authenticity, where clear feedback could be provided on levels of competence, for example 'skills mastery' where procedural skills were observed and 'ticked off' by educators.

Intersecting Foci? Learners' Survival Focus and Educators' Focus on Equipping Students with Agency

The transition programme was established to promote student agency in clinical education. The sessions were designed to help students develop a transferable set of skills relating to learning and communication in the clinical environment. Skills that were targeted included how to solicit feedback from educators and peers, how to self-assess performance, how to approach an educator if students felt a disconnect between what they had been taught and how they were being instructed, and how students could plan ahead to optimise self-care during a period characterised by change and a sharp learning trajectory.

Although students were able to identify these concepts as learning outcomes in the transition programme, they reported that they were thirsty for information on pragmatic issues, such as location of the physiotherapy clinic, car parking, and precise instructions about the expectations of student practice.

> Exactly what are the clinicians expecting us to do in that first week? (Student 3)
> I'm not sure what their expectations of us are, that's the other thing. I find them intimidating. I don't know if they expect us to be really good or expect us to be shocking... (Student 4)

Students in the focus group did not conceive a graded, incremental learning 'journey' and did not recognise that the clinicians would tailor learning experiences according to student's demonstrated capacity to work independently. This lack of student clarity exposed the lack of guidelines for clinical educators about what students should typically 'do' in the first 1–2 weeks in their clinical placement. For example, should students observe for day 1, and then be expected to perform a supervised history taking on day 2? The lack of explicit guidelines may be a function of the diversity in clinical practice (e.g. some placements are more complex than others, some environments carry higher stakes, etc.) and the assumption that learning is iterative and therefore less structure/guidance may be required for students in rotations 2 and 3. It may also be a result of the philosophy of 'tailored education' where the students' demonstrated knowledge, competence, and confidence will affect the learning/practice activity offered. Three outcomes have emerged from this research about students' apprehension about first placement performance expectations. First, 4th-year students have devised a list of domain-specific practice questions relating to each area of practice to better prepare year-3 students for the type of content knowledge required 'at their finger tips'. Second, each clinical site has posted a list of common conditions that are seen as part of practice, and third, focus group research is currently being conducted with clinical educators to establish how placements can be structured to promote better sequencing and scaffolding of student learning.

Students reported that their survival focus was twofold, reflecting the two perceived critical audiences in clinical education. They reported anxiety about looking the part with patients, and looking the part for clinical educators. Some students were concerned that clinical supervisors would detect their lack of knowledge/practice competence early in the placement:

> Will I be any good?... I'll open my mouth and the supervisors will know that I am not competent. (Student 1)

It was notable that students did not seem to use exam marks or OSCE (practical exam) results as a proxy for their likely clinical competence, thereby emphasising in their minds the difference, or disconnect, between performance in university-oriented activities and performance in authentic practice.

> So for example, for your OSCEs when you've had your simulated patients, the retired [physiotherapy] seniors, did you feel that talking to those patients felt different to talking to your peers? (Interviewer)
> Yep (Student 4) – But not to the same level as the actual patient, because you know that they're a physio, like they were good ... they do more what you expect, where as like [real] patients, you can't expect anything because they can do anything (Student 3)

This data suggests that the nature of briefing to prepare students for clinical practice needs to secure a balance between being informative, outlining the parameters for practice, including highlighting the pitfalls of novice practice, and remaining reassuring and positioning the students for capacity (e.g. you have the necessary platform of knowledge and skill to take on these new set of challenges).

4.5.1.2 Theme 2: Authenticity as the Driver for Learning

Student responses to both the questionnaire and the focus group questions indicated a strong awareness of the theory–practice divide. They were aware of the distinctly different challenges that they would confront working with 'real patients', in a 'real setting'. The stakes were seen to be higher, and to add to the anxiety of raising the stakes of practice, students were cognizant of the frequent and vigilant surveillance by clinical educators.

> So clinics are going to be about real patients (Student 1)
> Yeah, actually *doing* (Student 2)
> And heaps more responsibility (Student 1)
> And actual pathologies (Student 3)
> Like you do things here in pracs, like you'll do an anterior drawer test on someone that doesn't have an ACL problem. You've got no idea what you're actually feeling for. (Student 1)
> Like a neuro patient, we don't know what a hemiplegic limb actually feels like when you're lifting it. And if you are working on someone who's completely dependent on you .... It feels completely different to when we're doing it [on students] because I know you guys, I'm comfortable being around and touching you guys. (Student 2)
> The sort of practice that we do here seems to be insignificant compared to what we're going to be doing because like she said, it's like, I know Tom [student], I don't care if he falls. (Student 1)
> We all know in theory what it should be like but it will be very different in real life .... Our mere preconception of what it should be like is very different within each of us. (Student 4)

As described earlier in this chapter, the questionnaire results suggested that students privileged practical classes (technical skill development) as a key modality in preparing them for authentic practice. Students also raised the importance of immersion in clinical practice (including observation) as a way of better preparing them for workplace learning.

> It would make it a lot easier to practice effectively if we dealt with patients before. (Student 4)
> I think the most beneficial thing for [preparation for] clinics was the 9 hours or so of observation that we had last year. (Student 3)

Gordon et al.'s (2000) research on workplace transition emphasises the importance of learners 'hanging out' in their clinical environment, as a form of professional and institutional socialisation to 'smell the wards', observe the protocols, and listen to the language, prior to engaging in practice. The results of our study suggest that earlier exposure to clinical practice, which may include community-based settings, may provide students with a better understanding of practice expectations and target skills. Earlier exposure may also aid learners to see the relevance of what is sometimes labelled by students as 'softer' or 'iffy' or 'peripheral' components of curriculum. Additionally, clinical placements in year 3 and 4 may be better structured to allow for observation of, and reflection on, expert practice.

4.5.1.3 Theme 3: Facilitating Transition: Engagement with Canonical and Heuristic Knowledge

In the two focus groups, students suggested that they had come to appreciate two important functions in the transition programme curriculum. First, they reported the importance of learning the canonical knowledge of physiotherapy including conceptual content (e.g. anatomy, normative values for arterial blood gases), and the procedural skills to be able to practice effectively. Second, they reported that they learnt something of the heuristics (i.e. tricks of the trade) about what can go right and wrong in clinical practice, and the strategies to deal with complex clinical problems. Heuristics are often communicated or modelled informally and, typically, do not form part of explicit university-based curricula.

In line with Small et al.'s (2008) study, the data suggested that students appreciated the practical tips and experiences from 4th-year students. The informal 'storytelling' from lecturers was highly valued. An example of the praised 'storytelling' is shown below:

It was good to raise awareness [about palliative care], like ... giving us some strategies about this is a good way to cope, and this is how people ... or, here are some examples of things people say. (Student 2)

You know what was good was when Pauline [Lecturer] was telling us when she was in 3rd year she had a patient, and she was in the gym and she had to get them walking on bars or something and she got them to stand up and they had a DVT and ended up ... they died, right in front of her. And she was just sort of went through how she felt and then said that you know, what would you do if you were the supervisor and that happened to your student?, and we were like 'give them counselling' so she was like, 'well my supervisor sent me to the pub.' (Student 1)

This relaying of experience of the clinical interface appeared to be an important mechanism for helping students to understand context and ways in which their university-learned knowledge may be applied in practice. Another key theme, related to heuristics, was students' appreciation for tips on 'how to play the game' in clinical education. Figure 4.1 presents students' tips on transition to clinical education (Delany & Molloy, 2009); the most frequently presented tip was 'learn how to play the game,' that is, picking up on institutional and professional expectations and nuances, including negotiating the supervisory relationship.

Students stated that one of the best pieces of advice from the transition programme was about using the concept of 'reporting back' to clinical educators on their learning and performance. Focus group participants reported that at first, this 'reporting-back system' felt foreign as they did not commonly employ this as a mechanism in their university-based programme, and they feared it could be misrepresented as trying to impress their supervisors.

It was important to know that, and it was good reinforcing that it's ok to tell them [clinical educators] that I've gone and researched that. (Student 1)

The brown nosing! (Student 2)

Yes, the brown nosing because I wouldn't have done a whole lot of that. (Student 3)

Don't be shy to show your stuff- really talk to your supervisor and show them that you are working. (Student 1)

Constantly talk through your thought process with your supervisor. (Student 2)

I mean no one likes doing it, but I suppose, like, how much brown nosing, or reporting back, should we do? (Student 2)

Well it depends. I suppose the premise is that clinicians are busy and can't watch you all the time, so you are filling in the gaps and actually informing them what you have done for that day. (Interviewer)

Because it's not something we've done at uni before .... It's not something we are used to. (Student 3)

I suppose it does two things. It shows the educator that you're keen and interested and that you've done the work, but it also helps to unpack your clinical reasoning .... It's a form of transparency. (Interviewer)

In addition to students identifying the importance of canonical and heuristic-based knowledge, engagement in the learning activities was emphasised. Figure 4.2 summarises the three key elements that students identified as important in contributing to a successful transition to workplace learning. Canonical knowledge (including conceptual and procedural knowledge), and the revealing of 'tricks of the trade' were both seen as important. The ways that students were invited to engage in these forms of knowledge were also viewed as important. Students praised practical or interactive 'doing' exercises more than didactic-style lectures, and reported the importance of being able to see the *relevance* of the content they were being asked to learn. Specifically, they reported the value of contextually bound learning interventions such as case studies and practitioner 'war stories' and they identified that this signposting helped them to identify the knowledge provided as worth taking in. For example, students found 'scare tactics' signposting helpful, which may include a statement about the consequences of not knowing important material. An example of such educator signposting might include 'if you don't pick up a strength deficit, and sensation loss, you may miss a sinister pathology such as a spinal tumour.' Students were able to distil high-stakes knowledge/tasks from low-stakes knowledge/tasks on the basis of the consequences of knowing (or not knowing) that information. For students, stakes in learning were defined in relation

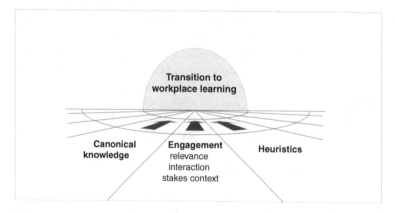

Fig. 4.2 Students' perceptions of key components driving transition

to anticipated effects on patient outcomes, the type of assessment applied (formative versus summative), and the potential for loss of face in front of two critical audiences: clinical educators and patients. The data suggested that students rapidly weigh up these factors when deciding how vigorously to engage with the curriculum offered.

The data from the questionnaire and focus group suggested that all three elements presented in Fig. 4.2 are important in designing a transition curriculum. The helpful heuristics identified by students rarely emerge from a formalised academic curriculum, and, in this sense, we suggest that such knowledge, and deliverers of knowledge (i.e. past students or clinical educators themselves) form part of a transition programme.

4.6 Conclusion and Recommendations

The transition programme was evaluated highly by physiotherapy students, with 90% of students who completed surveys agreeing or strongly agreeing that the learning objectives in the lectures/workshops were achieved. Students, in their appraisal of the 3-year academic curriculum and the transition programme, reported that the most valuable form of learning was practical sessions, with a focus on technical skill acquisition. This finding of the relative privileging of technical skill development is in alignment with previous studies on students' preparation for practice (Chumley et al., 2005; O'Brien, Cooke, & Irby, 2007; Prince et al., 2005; Small et al., 2008).

A key question that arises from this study is how can we convince and socialise students to the value of metacognitive learning so that they can develop a skill set equipping them for agency in workplace learning? Contemporary education literature advocates the importance of producing self-directed and reflective learners (Higgs et al., 2004; Kilminster & Jolly, 2000) but there is little evidence or instruction on how to achieve this goal (Baxter & Gray, 2001). The data from this study indicate that one of the constraints to students' engagement in this learning agenda is their quick judgement of 'iffy' or 'peripheral' content – viewed as removed from 'core business'. Utilising the advice of older students who have been working in the clinical environment and leaning on the heuristics and storytelling of clinicians may be two ways to reinforce relevancy and encourage learner engagement in the curriculum.

The transition programme was driven by the assumption that self-directed learning skills need to be scaffolded by educators in the academic setting, so that such skills become habit rather than an additional learning objective in the complex clinical environment. For example, students participated in an explicit lecture on reflective practice, and such metacognitive skills were drawn upon in sessions on educator and learner roles in clinical education, feedback, self-evaluation and assessment, and the sessions on learning preferences and leadership approaches. This curriculum contrasts to lectures in the first 2 years of the programme where there is a greater emphasis on appropriation of factual, biomedical knowledge. These 'meta' skills are likely to provide students with agency in their professional learning and to soften the sharp-edged transition between the university and clinical learning environments. In assisting students to identify potential stressors in the clinical learning environment, and through designing and practising strategies to meet such demands, it is hoped that transition programmes will help to free up cognitive capacity for workplace learning (Molloy, 2009). This chapter serves to untangle the multiple influences on preparation of students for clinical practice, and proposes practical approaches to help bridge university-based learning and clinical practice.

Storytelling and raising students' awareness of consequences of their knowledge (or lack of knowledge) on patient outcomes constitutes one way of selling important messages. Another way of turning what is seen as 'peripheral knowledge' into 'core knowledge' is to assess students' ability in reflection and metacognition (Delany & Molloy, 2009). Assessment can drive learning (Henderson et al., 2005), and students' comments supported that their attention was captured by the expectation of summative assessment. For example, educators could create discreet assessment criteria based on student ability to solicit feedback from the educator, or ability to self-evaluate performance. Such assessment would legitimise the expectations that these skills form part of artful practice. Finally, this research reinforces the importance of integration of curricular material, so that 'theme one' content (personal and professional practice) is framed within the context of clinical scenarios that include diagnostic and management skills. The results highlight the value that students ascribe to authenticity in learning. This search for experience-based learning may encourage educators to look for more creative teaching and learning opportunities in programmes, including earlier clinical immersion through community-based placements, video material of clinical assessments and treatments, and the use of low- and high-fidelity simulation.

While this programme has been designed to soften the interface between academic and workplace learning, we are not naïve to the concept that 'the only way to prepare for Rome, is Rome.' As one student aptly described 'I think that no matter what theory we get, we won't be prepared for it [practice].' A well-designed transition programme may help the student pack what they need for Rome, a map and some sturdy shoes for all types of terrain.

Acknowledgements This project forms part of a wider national and multidisciplinary research project investigating professional learning. The national project was led by Professor Stephen Billett from Griffith University and was supported by an Australian Council of Teaching and Learning Grant. We would also like to acknowledge Stephen Maloney for his expertise in helping to operationalise the transition programme in the Department of Physiotherapy, Monash University.

References

Ansari, W. (2003). Satisfaction trends in undergraduate physiotherapy education. *Physiotherapy*, *89*, 171–185.

Baxter, S., & Gray, C. (2001). The application of student-centred learning approaches to clinical education. *International Journal of Language and Communication Disorders, 36*(suppl. 2001), 396–400.

Billett, S. (2006). Constituting the workplace curriculum. *Journal of Curriculum Studies, 38,* 31–48.

Chumley, H., Olney, C., Usatine, R., & Dobbie, A. (2005). A short transitional course can help medical students prepare for clinical learning. *Family Medicine, 37,* 496–501.

Cupit, R. (1988). Student stress: An approach to coping at the interface between preclinical and clinical education. *Australian Journal of Education, 34,* 215–219.

Davis, M. H., & Harden, R. M. (1999). AMEE medical education guide no 15: Problem-based learning: A practical guide. *Medical Teacher, 21*(2), 130–140.

Delany, C., & Molloy, E. (2009). Critical reflection in clinical education: Beyond the swampy lowlands. In C. Delany & E. Molloy (Eds.), *Clinical education in the health professions* (pp. 3–24). Sydney: Elsevier.

Denniston, C., Molloy, E., & Nickson, W. (2010). Effective practice in clinical education: The supervisor's perspective. Manuscript submitted for publication.

Driessen, E., van Tartwijk, J., Overeem, K., Vermunt, J., & van der Vleuten, C. (2005). Conditions for successful reflective use of portfolios in undergraduate medical education. *Medical Education, 39,* 1230–1235.

Gordon, J., Hazlett, C., Ten Cate, O., Mann, K., Kilminster, S., Prince, K., et al. (2000). Strategic planning in medical education: Enhancing the learning environment for students in clinical settings. *Medical Education, 34,* 841–850.

Henderson, P., Ferguson-Smith, A., & Johnson, M. (2005). Developing essential professional skills: A framework for teaching and learning about feedback. *BMC Medical Education, 5,* 1–6.

Higgs, J., Richardson, B., & Abrandt Dahlgren, M. (2004). *Developing practice knowledge for health professionals.* Edinburgh: Butterworth Heinemann.

Keating, J., Dalton, M., & Davidson, D. (2009). Assessment in clinical education. In C. Delaney & E. Molloy (Eds.), *Clinical education in the health professions* (pp. 147–172). Sydney: Elsevier.

Kilminster, S., & Jolly, B. (2000). Effective supervision in clinical practice settings: A literature review. *Medical Education, 34,* 827–840.

Lave, J., & Wenger, E. (1991). *Situated learning: Legitimate peripheral participation.* Cambridge: University of Cambridge.

Le Maistre, C., & Pare, A. (2004). Learning in two communities: The challenge for universities and workplaces. *Journal of Workplace Learning, 16*(1/2), 44–52.

Molloy, E. (2009). Time to pause: Feedback in clinical education. In C. Delaney & E. Molloy (Eds.), *Clinical education in the health professions* (pp. 128–146). Sydney: Elsevier.

Molloy, E., & Clarke, D. (2005). The positioning of physiotherapy students and clinical supervisors in feedback sessions. *Focus on Health Professional Education: A Multi-disciplinary Journal, 7,* 79–90.

Moss, F., & McManus, I. (1992). The anxieties of new clinical students. *Medical Education, 26,* 17–20.

Neville, S., & French, S. (1991). Clinical education: Students' and clinical tutors' views. *Physiotherapy, 77,* 351–354.

O'Brien, B., Cooke, M., & Irby, D. M. (2007). Perceptions and attributions of third-year student struggles in clerkships: Do students and clerkship directors agree?. *Academic Medicine, 82,* 970–978.

Prince, K., Boshuizen, H., van der Vleuren, C., & Scherpbier, A. (2005). Students' opinions about their preparation for clinical practice. *Medical Education, 39,* 704–712.

Prince, K., Van De Wiel, M., Scherpbier, A., van Der Vleuten, C., & Boshuizen, H. (2000). A qualitative analysis of the transition from theory to practice in undergraduate training in a PBL-medical school. *Advances in Health Sciences Education, 5,* 105–116.

Radcliffe, C., & Lester, H. (2003). Perceived stress during undergraduate medical training: A qualitative study. *Medical Education, 37,* 32–38.

Rose, M., & Best, D. (2005). *Transforming practice through clinical education, professional supervision and mentoring.* Edinburgh: Elsevier.

Small, R., Soriano, R., Chietero, M., Quintana, J., Parkas, V., & Koestler, J. (2008). Easing the transition: Medical students' perceptions of critical skills required for the clerkships. *Education for Health, 20*(3), 1–9.

Strauss, A., & Corbin, J. (1998). *Basics of qualitative research: Techniques and procedures for developing grounded theory* (2nd ed.). London: Sage.

Van Gessel, E., Nendaz, M. R., Vermeulen, B., Junod, A., & Vu, N. V. (2003). Development of clinical reasoning from the basic sciences to the clerkships: A longitudinal assessment of medical students' needs and self-perception after a transitional learning unit. *Medical Education, 37*, 966–974.

Windish, D. M. (2000). Teaching medical students clinical reasoning skills. *Academic Medicine, 75*, 90.

Chapter 5
Optimising the Follow-through Experience for Midwifery Learning

Linda Sweet and Pauline Glover

5.1 Follow-through Experiences: Pedagogic and Curriculum Considerations

The provision of follow-through experiences for midwifery students is a requirement for meeting national midwifery curriculum standards and an important educational strategy for students to learn about continuity of care. This innovation is based on the experience where students engage with pregnant women through the period leading up to and immediately after the birth of their child or children. That is, the students follow-through with the woman during the antenatal, birth, and postnatal experience. Such experiences also constitute an innovation in the curriculum and pedagogic practices of midwifery educators and programmes. It is believed that the follow-through experience is a positive strategy for students to learn about continuity of care regardless of the availability of midwifery continuity of care models.

The follow-through experience has been mandated by the occupational accreditation authority. However, while some midwives believe the follow-through experience is a valuable learning interlude there are no evidence-based accounts to support this claim. This chapter takes up this challenge by describing and discussing the processes and outcomes of a research project aimed to identify the strengths and weaknesses of follow-through experiences as curriculum and pedagogic tools. In all, the study identifies positive aspects of the intended use of 'follow-throughs', as well as powerful but unintended contributions that might be described as the hidden curriculum. The findings from this qualitative study were derived from four focus groups and the analysis of reflective portfolios from past graduands. Three focus groups were conducted with a homogenous group of midwifery students from each year level (i.e. 1st, 2nd, 3rd year). The fourth focus group was conducted with midwifery academic staff. These data were analysed independently and then subjected to a thematic analysis to identify their potential and limitations as a form of learning

L. Sweet (✉)
Flinders University, Adelaide, SA 5042, Australia
e-mail: linda.sweet@flinders.edu.au

S. Billett, A. Henderson (eds.), *Developing Learning Professionals*, Professional and Practice-based Learning 7, DOI 10.1007/978-90-481-3937-8_5,
© Springer Science+Business Media B.V. 2011

support. The discussion that follows explores the usefulness of follow-throughs as a curriculum and pedagogic model to develop 'learning professionals'. Aspects of the intended curriculum – what was planned to be realised – will be highlighted along with components identified as the hidden curriculum – unintended learning outcomes – within the follow-through experience.

The chapter commences with an overview of midwifery education and the curriculum requirement of the follow-through experiences within it. Then, the intended use of follow-throughs is discussed, followed by an account of the kinds of knowledge that need to be learnt by midwives and how the follow-throughs can contribute to this knowledge development. The particular contributions are identified using extracts from the focus groups. A model of curriculum and pedagogic practices that support the effective use of follow-throughs is then proposed and discussed. The outcomes of this study are then summarised in the conclusion.

5.2 Midwifery and the Follow-through Experiences

Midwifery is a practice-based profession that involves caring for women and their families in the period from preconception through pregnancy to 6 weeks following the birth of the baby. A midwife is a person who works in partnership with women to give the necessary support, care, and advice during pregnancy, labour, and the postpartum period; to conduct births; and to provide care for the newborn and infant (World Health Organisation, 2009). Midwifery constitutes a long-standing occupation whose practices were often passed from generation to generation through storytelling and women supporting other women through the childbearing years (Affandi, 2002; Pairman, Pincombe, Thorogood, & Tracy, 2006; World Health Organisation, 2009). However, over time midwifery has evolved to become a regulated profession requiring education programmes that lead to the registration of practitioners. As a practice-based profession, midwifery requires practice-based experiences that can likely be acquired only through engagement in midwifery practice. To develop competence as autonomous practitioners, students of midwifery require experience in authentic practice environments that integrate with university-based learning.

Until 2002, midwifery preparation in Australia comprised a post-registration training programme building on a nursing qualification. However, since then midwifery education in Australia has seen marked changes, including the move from being a post-nursing registration certificate to an undergraduate degree in its own right. Consequently, the introduction of the 3-year Bachelor of Midwifery in Australia in 2002 brought key educational challenges about how best to prepare midwives who lack nursing qualification or experience. Regardless, midwifery education aims to achieve the development of the conceptual, procedural, and dispositional knowledge required for effective professional practice. Conceptual knowledge comprises 'knowing about' the concepts, facts, and propositions (Billett, 2001, p. 51) that relate to midwifery practice. Procedural knowledge is the 'knowing how' (Billett, 2001, p. 52) to practice as a midwife, while dispositional knowledge is about the values and attitudes (Billett, 2001, p. 53) related to midwifery, that is the 'knowing for' of professional practice.

One of the most significant curriculum and pedagogical changes in moving from a post-registration programme has been the introduction of the follow-through experience. The follow-through component of the programme is a continuity model for midwifery students whereby they are involved in pregnancy and childbirth in partnership with women. The follow-through is defined as follows:

> ... the ongoing midwifery relationship between the students and the woman from initial contact in early pregnancy through to the weeks immediately after the woman has given birth, across the interface between community and hospital settings. The intention of the follow-through experience is to enable students to experience continuity with individual women through pregnancy, labour and birth and the postnatal period, regardless of the availability of midwifery continuity of care models. (Australian College of Midwives Inc., 2006b)

It is expected that the follow-through experience will be an integrated learning experience across the 3 years of the midwifery programme. The midwifery peak professional body requires that a portion of practice-based learning can be achieved through follow-through experiences with students undertaking a minimum of 30 in the 3-year programme. The peak regulatory authorities, which include the Australian Nursing and Midwifery Council and Nursing and Midwifery boards at state and territory level, adopted the recommendations. The follow-through experience in Australia is unique to midwifery education throughout the world. The establishment of this integrated practice-based learning requirement has challenged educators to consider innovative ways to enact this pedagogical approach to develop agentic professionals. Given the contribution to learning that follow-throughs are expected to provide in midwifery education, it is necessary to describe the overall curriculum arrangements and the positioning of the follow-throughs in these arrangements.

5.3 Intended Follow-through Experience Curriculum

The follow-through experiences are a core component of the overall midwifery curriculum. The follow-through experience is afforded one-third of the total clinical practice hours across the 3-year programme. The three purposes that underpin the follow-through as a workplace-based experience are for students to: (i) engage with and reflect on the world of midwifery work; (ii) understand and develop their individual capacity for the profession; and (iii) understand the nuances of the many and diverse instances of midwifery practices and birthing women's trajectories. A number of processes are used to assist the student to realise the stated purposes, and these are now elaborated.

To effectively engage with and reflect on the world of midwifery, the student is required to recruit and manage their own caseload of follow-throughs that meet the minimum requirements as stated in the curriculum. Students are then required to write a brief reflection on an aspect of their experiences at the completion of the follow-through. This is documented in a reflective portfolio for summative assessment. This 'write-up' includes an introduction to the woman and her family, a brief reflection of the student's understanding of the experience of pregnancy, birth, and postnatal period and a statement about what meaning this experience has had for their learning about midwifery. Students are provided with an example of how to write these experiences to give some structure and prevent an unrealistic word length. These reflective write-ups of the follow-through experience are the only assessment of this work-integrated learning model.

To develop canonical occupational concepts and procedures, the intent of the follow-through is for students to move from observation to participation in care of the childbearing woman, in a variety of midwifery practice settings over the 3 years of study. The overall curriculum aims for the Bachelor of Midwifery is that in the 1st year the students gain an awareness of midwifery practice. In the 2nd year it is intended that they develop their midwifery practice and by the 3rd year they consolidate their midwifery practice, as competent novice practitioners. The provision of practice experiences through the follow-through provides this pathway for development. Consequently, in the 1st year students observe clinical practice in a midwifery setting; in 2nd year they actively participate in providing midwifery care under direct supervision; and in the 3rd year they engage in the activities that develop the capacities to practice autonomously as a midwife.

An understanding of the nuances of the many and diverse practice settings is developed as students are exposed to a variety of models of care, as well as differing practices of midwives, obstetricians and general medical practitioners while undertaking their required follow-throughs. These may be across both public and private settings. The curriculum intent is for the student to gain experience of women-centred care, whereby the focus is on the woman, her health needs, and her expectations and aspirations (Australian College of Midwives Inc., 2006a). The follow-through experience promotes this through aligning the student with the woman rather than with a care provider in whichever model through which the woman is receiving her care.

During the development of the Bachelor of Midwifery, academic staff formulated a definition of the follow-through, however, the definition offered no insights into the actual practice of engaging in follow-throughs. Furthermore, there was no readily available literature about this activity as a clinical experience model. The expectations of students in these experiences were drafted with little understanding about how the students should be guided to partake in the experience; that is there was a limited pedagogical basis. The follow-through experiences are essentially not facilitated. With little guidance and no facilitation the students' active engagement is very much self-directed. The students' involvement with 'hands on' clinical tasks is variable depending on the students' year level, experience, and personal agency, primary care providers, and women's preferences. Therefore, the effectiveness of the follow-through experience is dependent on the ability of the midwifery student to recruit pregnant women and then establish and maintain partnerships with women and the care providers over the duration of the follow-through experience.

Furthermore, the academic staff have no control over the variety of experiences a student is afforded, or their exposure to variables such as models of care, primary care providers, duration of contact with women, good or bad role models, and individual personalities. The learning achieved in the follow-through experience is student-led, student-controlled, and student-directed and therefore the follow-through experience has the potential to greatly influence the development of agency in the student. And conversely, the agency of the student has the potential to greatly impact the learning outcomes of the follow-through experience.

While the follow-through experience is one portion of the clinical experiences across the 3-year programme of study, it is the only clinical midwifery exposure for students in the 1st year of the course. While other clinical experience is gained in nursing settings in the 1st year, the follow-through experience is specific to maternity care and childbearing women. In the 2nd and 3rd year of the programme, students are required to attend midwifery settings in blocks of time, working under direct supervision of midwives in addition to their follow-through experiences.

5.4 Developing Learning Professionals

A qualitative research approach was undertaken to investigate the intent and enactment of the follow-through experience as a pedagogic approach. Focus groups were conducted with 1st-, 2nd-, and 3rd-year current midwifery students in their year groups to explore their perceptions and experiences of the follow-through portion of the curriculum. The focus group of midwifery academic staff explored their perceptions of the follow-through portion of the curriculum. In addition to these focus groups, reflective portfolios recording follow-through experiences across the 3 years of the programme were collected from graduand students. These data were individually and collectively subject to thematic analysis to identify the follow-through experience's potential and limitations as a form of learning support.

This research has demonstrated there are many ways that professional learning can be supported and/or hindered in the follow-through experience as a midwifery practice-based learning model. The key themes that emerged from this research that contribute to supporting professional learning through the follow-through experience include the student: developing awareness of the role of the midwife; developing their personal midwifery identity; skill development; development from lay to professional language; and progress from description to reflection. It is important to acknowledge that learning in the follow-through was also hindered by some negative experiences such as the emotional impact, time commitment, financial cost, and personal safety. However, our primary focus here is to demonstrate how midwifery learning is optimised through the follow-through experience. This is particularly worth noting because in many ways the midwifery students epitomised what is being asked of students in work-integrated learning arrangements, that is to engage actively, professionally, and conscientiously in professionally premised activities. Yet, while this can lead to rich learning, it can also constitute experiences that have powerful personal impacts.

As a means to demonstrate the powerful learning afforded by the follow-through, the following discussion is based on the intent of workplace learning models, that is, the development of conceptual, procedural, and dispositional knowledge for effective occupational practice. These different forms of knowledge are described in detail with examples of how the follow-through assists students in the development of both the intended and the hidden curriculum. Examples from the data are presented as evidence for the discussion. Recommendations for optimising the follow-through as a learning model are then proposed.

5.5 Conceptual Midwifery Knowledge

Conceptual knowledge is the development of facts, information, propositions, assertions, and concepts for practice and is developed over time from integration between theory and practice. Conceptual knowledge is achieved in increasing complexity from simple factual knowledge (e.g. names of pieces of equipment, tools or workplace procedures) through to deeper levels of conceptual knowledge (Billett, 2001). Complex conceptual midwifery knowledge, the 'knowing about' midwifery, develops from a deep understanding of the concepts, facts and propositions of midwifery practice. The development of this requires the student to be thoughtful and reflective on their experiences in both the university and workplace-based setting. Therefore, conceptual midwifery knowledge is not achievable from theory or classroom-based learning alone. A 1st-year student commented:

> I guess the class learning ... it's theory, you know and it's discussion and it's ideas. ... there is a lot of great chats that happens in some of our labs, at some of our pracs, but when you're out in it you're seeing it happen, it's a real life process, what the midwives are doing. (1st-year focus group)

This research has shown that in the 1st year, conceptual midwifery knowledge is developed through the triad relationship in the workplace between the student, the childbearing woman, and the maternity healthcare providers, and underpinned by their university-based learning. The follow-through optimises this conceptual learning through early exposure to midwifery practice, which enables the student to experience concepts such as continuity of care and women-centred care. Factual and propositional knowledge is achieved only at a basic, almost lay level in the 1st year as driven by the curriculum. However, by the completion of the 3 years of the programme this factual and propositional knowledge becomes highly sophisticated through the continued experiences the follow-through affords. The continuity of care that the follow-through provides is the vehicle for 'knowing about' midwifery in a more meaningful way. The traditional clinical block placement provides fragmented care and therefore limited opportunity for midwifery students to get to know the woman and her needs during pregnancy, birth, and the postnatal period.

The follow-through enabled students to recognise the many and varied contexts in which midwifery work is done. Students recognise the value and importance of continuity of care for the woman and the midwife. It was found that through the follow-through students learnt about the key tenets of the: (i) value and importance of continuity of care; (ii) continuity of carer for the birthing woman; and (iii) continuity of learning/preceptor for the midwifery student. It is the continued contact with the pregnant woman that the follow-through experience affords that promotes this learning.

> Yeah, because you're seeing the whole range of different models, different hospitals. You're seeing different approaches and in some ways, I suppose, I imagine when you're on clinical you're under the supervision of a particular person and doing things their way; you're not so woman focused. Whereas when you're sitting with a woman and hearing her comments before and after the appointments, then you're really looking at it from her point of view. (1st-year focus group)

The key difference between the traditional block placement of work-based experiences and the follow-through experience is the alignment of the student with the woman as opposed to the care provider. As these students describe, the follow-through experience provided them perspective on maternity care very different from those provided by the traditional models.

In addition, four key areas of learning about the concept of 'continuity' were generated through the follow-through experience. These were: (i) the importance of learning from birthing women; (ii) learning from engaging with midwives; (iii) dependence on relationships with the birthing women and midwives; and (iv) recognition that the follow-through experience is not a realistic model of midwifery continuity of care.

> So what experience you get will be dependent on that relationship you build with the woman and then in a way if you can convey that relationship with the midwives who you work with, the obstetrician, so they know that you've got their confidence and can do some of the procedures under guidance and stuff. If you don't build up that relationship with a woman or she changes her mind then all bets are off. (3rd-year focus group)

The ability to develop a meaningful relationship between the student and the woman was integral to the learning experiences the student was afforded. Procedural learning in particular was very much dependent not only on the relationships the student built with the woman, but also with the midwife or lead-care provider. Students spoke candidly about the value of time in developing these relationships – the more they could meet or speak with mothers, midwives, and other staff related to the delivery of healthcare the better their relationship.

Conceptual knowledge development is achieved through thoughtful reflection on practice. This research has demonstrated that early in the programme, students do not have the ability to effectively reflect. Over time as they progress through the course and their knowledge and understanding about midwifery increases, their skill to reflect broadens considerably and they move from description to critical reflection. This shift is significant for midwifery students in increasing their capacity to become agentic learners. This ability as a reflective practitioner is achieved over time in the follow-through experience and is evident through the written reflections incorporated in the portfolio assessment. The reflective write-ups clearly demonstrated that students were comfortable and confident in describing their experiences.

The students' ability to reflect and therefore develop conceptual midwifery knowledge improved over time and students were able to identify 2nd year as a turning point for this process. A 2nd-year student reflected:

> I think they'd be completely different write ups, I'm just assuming that my write ups would be completely different because I really know now what I'm talking about for one thing. (2nd-year focus group)

Through the follow-through experience students were able to demonstrate the development of conceptual midwifery knowledge. They were able to recognise the varied contexts in which midwifery work occurs, and identify the learning they achieved from working with the women and midwives. This conceptual knowledge development was enhanced as they further developed their reflective practice. Integrated with the development of their conceptual knowledge was the identification of procedural knowledge for midwifery practice.

5.6 Procedural Knowledge

Midwifery as a practice-based profession requires the development of procedural knowledge in order to acquire the skills for safe, competent midwifery practice. 'Knowing how' to practice as a midwife is more than the ability to undertake procedural skills in isolation. While individual skills may be able to be rote learnt, or learnt in simulated settings, procedural knowledge is more than this and requires the student to apply their skills in the context of midwifery practice.

The follow-through experience provides a range of opportunities for procedural knowledge development. However, this is often not in synchrony with the academic curriculum, as during the follow-throughs students are exposed to skills and procedures in practice that they may not yet have learned in the university setting. Procedural learning in the follow-through commences with the recruitment of the students' first woman, when they begin to learn about pregnancy and midwifery care. Not surprisingly, given their concern to be competent in their new practice, much of the student effort through the follow-throughs was focused on procedural learning. Furthermore, there was a strong desire for the development of the procedures required to effectively assist the woman to birth her baby. In this way it constitutes a birth centric enacted curriculum, and appeared to be experienced by students as such. However, there were unplanned outcomes. For instance, there was learning that occurred outside of the preferred sequence for developing midwifery competence. Students were exposed to normal and abnormal presentations without the concomitant factual knowledge and skills. These new and 'exciting' aspects of practice were highly valued by students.

> Mostly the new things that pop up and there's a lot of them now and hopefully they'll get less and less but yeah all of the things that are exciting that I haven't seen before. (1st-year focus group)

Students were either asked to or requested to be involved in procedures about which their understanding may have been quite limited. Certainly, the emphasis on procedural learning went beyond the intended observation of practice in the early phases of their development. The students craved task learning associated with 'midwifery work', and provided rich and enthusiastic accounts of their 'first experiences', which overrode some of the staged intentions for the midwifery programme. Certainly, the students used their expanding midwifery skills as evidence of and a proxy for their developing knowledge and ability as midwives.

Students reported the follow-through as a place for opportunistic learning. Some students quickly developed confidence and agency in embracing these opportunities and to learn from these opportunities, while others students would only observe until first having the university-based instruction and learning. Therefore, the follow-through resulted in some students undertaking skills and procedures without the conceptual knowledge that underpins their practice. Students identified the challenge of developing their procedural knowledge in the follow-through experience.

> It's hard, it's like she said, in 1st year you don't have the skills, so it's good to be able to practice the skills and get your confidence up in that way. Second year you do have the skills but you also don't need as much practice because you're getting that in the clinical area. (2nd-year focus group)

The kinds of opportunities afforded students for procedural development were dependent on the relationship the students developed with the healthcare providers and their willingness to teach the student. Therefore, the follow-through offers students the opportunity to extend their procedural knowledge; it is not the foundation for initial development.

> I've been really lucky. I've had midwives who've just spilled all their knowledge out at me and wanted to ... even things beyond .... (1st-year focus group)

Students who embraced these learning opportunities found them beneficial in building their confidence. They were able to see the procedure and its place in practice, be exposed to procedural rules and guidelines in practice, learn the procedure under guidance, and then integrate and reflect on their practice of the procedure once covering the procedure at the university. Through the authenticity of the learning, this approach greatly enhanced students' self-directedness as learner and their agency. The out-of-synchrony learning was a positive contribution to the students' engagement with the learning and integration of their knowledge over time.

> I think you're just constantly building up your own little reservoir of knowledge. I mean I know now I sit with the follow-throughs and just the questions I'm asking them are completely different than what they used to be before I knew what I was talking about. (2nd-year focus group)

A disadvantage of the follow-through experience for procedural knowledge development is the lack of repetition and continuity of supervision and therefore formative feedback on progress. Students often commented that the traditional block placement allowed them to focus on specific sets of skills more effectively than the follow-through did, however, such a focus compartmentalises midwifery proce-dural knowledge. The follow-through experience allowed students the opportunity to practice and consolidate their procedural knowledge in the context of holistic care with the woman at the centre of events. In this context, the follow-throughs enabled practice in the safety of a known relationship with the women whereby the student was encouraged by the women to 'have a go'. This known relationship, how-ever, was a disadvantage when it came to intimate procedures for some students, as their relationship with the woman was a personal one more than a professional one. Students expressed unease at subjecting the woman to their incompetence or devel-oping competence for intimate procedures such intrapartum vaginal examinations as they had built a close and trusting personal relationship.

The development of procedural knowledge was evident as students were exposed to midwifery practice through the follow-through experience. They identified the development of midwifery skills which became more sophisticated over time. Acculturation to the clinical setting occurs as the students have more exposure to midwifery practice and this leads to the identification of the development of their dispositional knowledge.

5.7 Dispositional Knowledge

Dispositional knowledge relates to the values and attitudes required for midwifery practice and the ability to 'be' a midwife. The follow-through experience provides the midwifery student with the opportunity to observe midwifery practice; reflect on their own values, attitudes, affect, and interest; and establish their own midwifery identity. The follow-through experience is a successful model to assist the student to develop and demonstrate dispositional knowledge and professional boundaries. Students come to the programme of study with their own perceptions and attitudes about whom and what a midwife is or should be, and where and how they want to practice. The active participation in the follow-through experience is challenging these preconceptions and attitudes over time which assists students to clarify and develop their own professional midwifery identity. Developing the awareness of the role of the midwife begins at the commencement of the course of study. Students' preconceived idea of the role of the midwife may or may not be accurate and is challenged through both the classroom learning and the clinical experience. While this 1st-year student has had her preconceived ideas challenged, the follow-through offered greater opportunities for reflection on the midwife's role and her future place in healthcare.

> I'm learning what a midwife's job really is because I came in with all my ideas and as a woman excited about birth in the community .... I'm actually seeing what they're doing with their work which is a big – it's a new experience .... (1st-year focus group)

The follow-through experience provides the midwifery student with the oppor-tunity to understand the totality of the woman's experiences. Decisions and nego-tiations that confront birthing women, and how these may vary, not only because of health-related factors, but also through those associated with their family, economic, and social standing, were further influences on the students' learning. Hence, the premises for becoming an advocate for birthing women were afforded by the follow-through experience. The fact that students were exposed to diverse healthcare professionals through the follow-through experience, enabled them to reflect on, and begin to construct, their own philosophy of practice, and hence their own midwifery identity. Through reflection on their own experiences from the follow-through experience and from their exposure to midwifery role models, students were able to identify how they would like to practice as a midwife.

> Well I guess firstly you learn the way you'd ideally like to work . . . after you have studied.
> (2nd-year focus group)

While the follow-through experience provided a range of role modelling opportunities, the students were left to identify good and bad role models for themselves. Early in the programme this was based on a very limited knowledge of the professional role. The exposure to a range of different practices by midwives, ancillary, and related healthcare practitioners was instrumental in the development of students' professional roles. Opportunities to participate in increased clinical care and decision-making became evident across the 3 years of the course and would appear to be a significant advantage of the follow-through experience.

The follow-through experience engages midwifery students in partnership with women from the beginning of the 3-year programme of study. While the students are provided the international definition of the midwife, in the 1st semester this is an esoteric concept and it is not until they are exposed to practice through the follow-through experience that they can identify its true meaning and begin to establish their own midwifery identity that meets the requirements of the international definition of a midwife.

It is clear that the intent of the follow-through experience as part of the wider curriculum is to produce an agentic professional who will acquire the midwifery knowledge and skills to meet the requirements necessary for registration as a midwife. The students are able to focus their learning on the meaning of pregnancy, birth, and postnatal experience for the woman while at the same time developing their own professional identities and dispositions. Students move from developing an awareness of practice to reflection and immersion in practice over the 3 years of study. The curriculum document clearly states the prescribed number of follow-through experiences to be completed, the time allocated for completion, and the assessment required. As with any curriculum there are discrepancies between the intended curriculum as set out by the institution, and the enacted or taught curriculum. These discrepancies occur due to the nuances of the workplace setting and people within it and the hidden curriculum. 'The hidden curriculum is the informal learning in which students engage and which is unrelated to what is taught' (Dent & Harden, 2005, p. 12). This research has shown that the follow-through experience as a curriculum model is not immune to this phenomena and the following section discusses what has been identified as the hidden curriculum in the follow-through experience.

5.8 Hidden Curriculum

As discussed above, the intended curriculum of the follow-through experience is for students to engage with and reflect on the world of midwifery work; to understand and develop their individual capacity for the profession; and to understand the nuances of the many and diverse practice settings. As demonstrated from the results of this research these are all achieved throughout the follow-through experience to varying degrees and at varying stages of the 3-year programme. Additionally, this component of the wider curriculum is supplemented with traditional block placements of clinical practice to enable consolidation of knowledge and skills in the clinical context. There are, however, components learnt in the follow-through experience which could be argued are within the realm of a hidden curriculum. This includes an understanding and development of the students' own personal and professional boundaries. To account for and manage these perceived boundaries midwifery students acknowledged the development of their personal agency in managing their follow-through experience load, and their development as strategic learners. In the beginning, often students give too much of themselves, physically, emotionally, and socially, and, over time, learn not to do this.

The follow-through experience requires students to recruit and follow-through 30 pregnant women across the 3-year course of study. This quantum of follow-through experiences is a daunting task, and midwifery students initially seek women from all possible networks including their friends, family, local community, and health services. As such, women are recruited into the follow-through relationship – in some instances – from a prior relationship with the student. Furthermore, as this is their only exposure to midwifery practice and maternity care in 1st year, students immersed themselves in the experience of pregnancy, birth, and midwifery practice, craving significant frequency and active involvement with pregnant women and midwives. Midwifery students described wanting to offer women something more than being a mere bystander in the experience but struggling to locate a role for themselves when they did not have the knowledge and experience as a health professional. Midwifery students clearly articulated a pattern of beginning the follow-through experience wanting to be a 'friend' or support person for the women. To this end, at the commencement of the midwifery follow-through experience, students were forming personal relationships with women on a level of friendship. As the students undertook a number of follow-through experiences, the time commitment and emotional involvement became apparent and students began to think and behave as strategic learners.

Students learnt very quickly that the follow-through experience was a time-unlimited undertaking, and they could put into the experience as much or as little time as they desired. Furthermore, this time management needed to take into consideration personal, family, and social commitments in addition to the needs of their study and the follow-through experience. This open-ended time commitment of the 30 follow-throughs over the 3-year programme enabled the realisation and generation of capacities by the students for being agentic and strategic in their engagement with these learning activities. Once the initial novelty of involvement in the follow-through experience passed, students became very strategic in recruiting women that they considered would be less demanding on their time, and more productive for meeting assessment requirements in relation to the volume of follow-through experiences required. Women pregnant for the second or subsequent time, those who had a history of quick labour or were advanced in their pregnancy became priority recruitment targets for students. This was a deliberate and targeted approach by the students to minimise their time in meeting course requirements. This resulted in fostering an attitude of favouring a fast birth and efficient time management, rather than taking the women-centred philosophy espoused within the programme.

Along with the strategic recruitment students learnt, came the identification and ability to maintain a professional-level relationship and setting of boundaries around the follow-through relationship between student and pregnant woman.

> It's taught me how to build a personal and then know how to separate it into a professional. I've learnt the difference between having a personal and a professional relationship. Its take a long time and a few mistakes along the way. But I've learnt that. (3rd-year focus group)

Therefore, the ability to develop professional rather than personal relationships changed the dynamics of the follow-through relationships students developed with women from personal to professionally bounded ones.

A component of the students' development of personal agency as a professional and learner was their experience of the follow-through experience as a learning model. The students arrived in the workplace aligned with the pregnant women and as a guest in the healthcare setting. The attitude and approach they were afforded by the health professionals made a significant impact on their perception of the follow-through experience as a learning experience. The relationships developed with the healthcare professionals became context-dependent and the students' experience was dependent on whether the midwife or doctor was a 'good teacher' and guided their learning or not. At times the learning was 'hidden' as the midwifery students were actively engaged in tasks but with no concomitant knowledge or understanding of the consequences of what they were doing. Students identified the limited support that the follow-through model afforded them when out in the workplace.

> That's probably more about working with different midwives and each person you work with has a different approach to how they want to do things, how things should be done. So you're really at the mercy of not your learning and what we learn at uni, but how each midwife practices throughout that follow-through experience. (3rd-year focus group)

Students became very aware of the impact of the facilitation of learning on the follow-through model and their dependence on the healthcare providers to afford them opportunities to learn, and provide expert guidance and opportunities to reflect on practice and develop that deep conceptual knowledge. The behaviours and norms of the health professionals became another component of the hidden curriculum as students learnt who to approach and who not to approach for their learning. It is recognised that good and bad professional role models exist in both follow-through experience and block clinical placements. The results of this study have added to the evidence that the hidden curriculum is dynamic and recursive – and can have both positive and negative influences on learning and the development of professionalism (Phillips, 2009).

5.9 A Conceptual Model for the Follow-through Experience

Canonical knowledge consists of the integration of all three forms of knowledge – conceptual, procedural, and dispositional. Given the enactment of these forms of knowledge development in the follow-through experience, there are a range of considerations for how these learning experiences might be maximised before, during, and after they have occurred.

5.9.1 Before the Follow-through Experience

At the commencement of the Bachelor of Midwifery and prior to the engagement with follow-through experience, it is beneficial that the following strategies be implemented to optimise student learning. First, students should be broadly prepared for the kinds of concepts, practices, and language that they are likely to encounter in their initial experiences. They need to be made aware of the boundaries of their professional practice and have the opportunity to consider ways in which these might be best managed. Exposure to a range of scenarios that the midwifery student might face will provide opportunities for the development of procedural capacities to negotiate real life experiences and actively engage students. Role playing ways in which to approach women and recruit them for the follow-through experience, and ways in which to bring closure to the relationship, is an example of exposure to such scenarios. Also, a level of proficiency in basic procedural skills such as blood pressure measurement, abdominal palpation, and foetal heart auscultation will assist the midwifery student to realise their desire to engage in midwifery work, but in ways that are appropriate and helpful. Educating students about the reality of midwifery work being more than the birthing process may well help them to identify the professional role of the midwife and position their follow-through experiences within the broader scope of midwives' work.

Given the independent nature of this set of experiences, reflective practice is essential to capture and enrich the learning. Midwifery students need to be prepared to reflect on practice and therefore require assistance with understanding the difference between description and reflection and how best to use these for learning. In order to enhance students' reflective practice it is suggested that these be introduced early in the curriculum, to inform students about what they are and how to do them. Providing examples or prompts of reflection on practice does enhance the midwifery students' progress to being a reflective practitioner. Heightened awareness of the concept of reflection was evident in this research from 2nd year onward, following formal assessment of a reflective essay. Providing a more formal structure for reflection on practice early in the curriculum should optimise learning. This can be achieved through aligning the structure of reflection with the intended curriculum content for each year level.

The organisation of follow-through experiences is likely to be enhanced by structured guidelines that contain the intended learning for the midwifery student. The guidelines need to be communicated to the health professionals with whom the students interact. The guidelines need, first, to contain clear instructions on how to engage the students in the recruitment and care of the woman, and closure of the follow-through. Second, for the health professionals supporting student learning the guidelines need to clearly state the intended curriculum for each year level. This will ensure consistency, potentially minimise out-of-sync learning, and assist with the development of relationships and professional boundaries. To maximise the variety and breadth of experiences midwifery students are exposed to during the follow-throughs, consideration should be given to encouraging students to experience different models and contexts of care.

As a core component of the curriculum, the follow-through experience needs to be effectively embedded in the assessment processes: to increase interaction with the experience; to improve conscious learning; and to give recognition to the time commitment from both the midwifery student and the woman. Integral to curricula improvement is the reconsideration of quality of learning from individual follow-throughs rather than the focus achieving a quantity of 30 across the programme of study as is currently required by the registering authorities. Structuring the follow-through experience prior to the midwifery student recruiting their first follow-through woman will go some way to assist in optimising their learning. Attention to supporting the midwifery students' learning during and after the follow-through experience is also required.

5.9.2 During the Follow-through Experience

During the follow-through experience it is important that midwifery students are given the opportunity to reflect on and in action, asking questions of the women and care providers in order to assimilate their knowledge with the care provided. This is the time when conceptual, procedural, and dispositional knowledge begin to integrate, and improved facilitation of learning by health professionals is one way to achieve this. Authentic learning is achieved when the midwifery student is afforded active participation in a 'hands-on' role as a care provider and not just the woman's companion or observer. Being afforded such participation requires the student to be viewed as a member of the healthcare team, and not just an appendage of the woman. Students can encourage this shift by actively involving themselves in the provision of care, and seeking advice and feedback from the woman and the care providers about their role. Incorporating workplace-based assessment practices is one way in which such involvement can be formalised. Midwifery student learning is further optimised through effective positive role modelling.

Guided learning is dependent on the care providers, the context of care, the environment in which the care providers are operating, and the relationships developed between student, woman, and healthcare professional. These factors are components of the hidden curriculum and unable to be controlled within the follow-through experience. Therefore, the development of effective relationships between individuals from within the educational intuition and the healthcare organisations may go some way to positively influence the guided learning for students. This guidance along with integration of experiences supports the construction of the midwifery students' canonical knowledge.

Engagement with the follow-through experience is a 'hot action' learning process, which requires on-the-spot reflection in the midst of rapid, ongoing action (Hoffman & Donaldson, 2004) and is the exciting component for students. However, learning is optimised if this is followed up by 'cold action' learning whereby students are guided through a process of debriefing and critical reflection on these experiences to identify and maximise learning (Hoffman & Donaldson, 2004).

5.9.3 After the Follow-through Experience

After the follow-through experiences it is important that students have the opportunity to share their experiences with peers and also with their lecturers. This sharing of follow-through experiences can have a powerful impact upon all students' learning, as this can expose midwifery students to a range of childbearing women and midwifery care. Students may be exposed to a variety of physiological, psychological, social, emotional, religious, and cultural circumstances for women, and to a range of actual pregnancy and birthing situations. So, opportunities for students to reflect upon and share their experiences with other students and lecturing staff likely provide a rich base to maximise the learning gained from these experiences. Such opportunities lend themselves to a shared construction of knowledge among students. This reflective time should be facilitated by a midwife because they have the canonical knowledge to guide students through the process of reflection and development of conceptual knowledge. These opportunities may focus on issues of practice, learning, and delineations of professional engagement. The very comprehensive nature of the follow-through experience sees it as being a central device for the development of midwifery skills and identity, and warrants integrating effectively within the overall midwifery curriculum.

Given the continuous nature of students' engagement in follow-through experience, many of the 'teacherly' concerns will need to be exercised before and during the experiences. Yet, throughout the follow-through experience there is a need to regularly engage students in reflecting upon their experiences. This will allow them to focus on the development of their canonical knowledge and their capacity as a midwife, including their ability to separate personal and professional boundaries. This reflection will assist the development of their agency as a learner operating in autonomous circumstances.

Implementing this conceptual model will go some way to optimise midwifery student learning in the follow-through experience. This conceptual model could be applied to any profession using a continuity of care model similar to that espoused by the follow-through experience.

5.10 Conclusions

The follow-through experience is a useful clinical learning opportunity as initial preparation of professional practitioners and offers the development of canonical knowledge for the smooth transition into practice. While the current follow-through experience goes some way to develop agentic professionals, our project has highlighted how these clinical experiences can be further enhanced to benefit the students' learning. Furthermore, a range of implications for teaching and learning arose from these findings, particularly for experiential and work-integrated learning. These included the importance of finding ways before, during, and after workplace-based experiences such as the follow-through experience to support midwifery students. Given the nature of midwifery work and the follow-through experience these experiences may go on over time and in locations and circumstances which are not always easily managed. Preparation and consideration of ways to support learning before, during, and after is crucial. By knowing what is expected and being prepared students will be enabled to effectively participate in and learn from the follow-through experience. It is also clear that the follow-through experiences provide exposure to both good and bad professional role models. Learning through these experiences needs to be guided to ensure midwifery students identify the 'good' role models to assist in the development of canonical knowledge. This highlights the importance of preparing both clinicians and students for follow-through practice and the importance of reflection on practice. Moreover, and quite specific to this midwifery programme, is a concern to enhance the quality of the experiences of the entire birthing process rather than emphasise the quantum of those experiences. That is, reducing the number of follow-throughs from the current level of 30 may well be a very sound pedagogical approach to improve the quality of the overall learning outcomes. In all, it was concluded that follow-through experience helps develop students' agentic learning capacities as previously shown.

Acknowledgements The authors wish to acknowledge the support provided by the Australian Learning and Teaching Council.

References

Affandi, B. (2002). Injectable contraceptives: A worldwide perspective. [Editorial] *The Journal of Family Planning and Reproductive Health Care, 28*(1), 3–5.

Australian College of Midwives Inc. (2006a). *Philosophy statement.* Canberra, ACT: Author.

Australian College of Midwives Inc. (2006b). *Standards for the accreditation of Bachelor of Midwifery Education programs leading to initial registration as a midwife in Australia.* Canberra, ACT: Author.

Billett, S. (2001). *Learning in the workplace: Strategies for effective practice*. Crows Nest, NSW: Allen & Unwin.

Dent, J., & Harden, R (Eds.). (2005). *A practical guide for medical teachers* (2nd ed.). Edinburgh: Elsevier.

Hoffman, K., & Donaldson, J. (2004). Contextual tensions of the clinical environment and their influence on teaching and learning. *Medical Education, 38,* 448–454.

Pairman, S., Pincombe, J., Thorogood, C., Tracy, S. (Eds.). (2006). *Midwifery preparation for practice*. Sydney: Churchill Livingstone.

Phillips, C. (2009). Student portfolios and the hidden curriculum on gender: Mapping exclusion. *Medical Education, 43,* 847–853.

World Health Organisation (2009). Nursing and midwifery human resources for health. Global standards for the initial education of professional nurses and midwives. Geneva: Author.

Chapter 6
A Considered Curriculum for Preparing Human Services Practitioners: Structuring Circles of Learning and Change

Jennifer Cartmel

6.1 Preparing Human Service Practitioners: A Considered Curriculum

Students who undertake practicum in human services and social work find themselves in a range of settings with a diverse range of people that are quite novel to them and, sometimes, can be quite confronting (Chenoweth & McAuliffe, 2005). The nature of human service work entails supporting and empowering individuals, families, and communities. Practitioners in this field are typically focused on working 'towards combating injustices that beset people, communities and entire nations because of oppression, violence, exploitation or simply the denial of basic human needs' (Chenoweth & McAuliffe, 2005, p. 32). Sometimes, this work involves engaging with individuals and families who are experiencing challenging and adverse circumstances, which may be beyond the experiences and even expectations of novice practitioners. Therefore, the challenges for these practitioners can include interacting with individuals and groups who are vulnerable and feeling pressured emotionally, yet may express their circumstances in confronting behaviour. Human service students often refer to being ill-prepared for the challenges such as these that they experience in human service field placements (Cartmel & Thomson, 2007). It follows, therefore, that an adequate preparation for students entering the work-based learning environment requires a carefully constructed curriculum for these novice practitioners that allows them to be both effective in their work and retain their sense of self through that work.

In considering these issues, this chapter discusses the delicate balance in curriculum design and teaching practice – the considered curriculum – that is essential to guide and support students' experience during their practicums. It describes strategies that seek to engage students in a straightforward critically reflective appraisal of professional issues that they may encounter and to which they need respond.

J. Cartmel (✉)
Griffith University, Brisbane, QLD, Australia
e-mail: j.cartmel@griffith.edu.au

S. Billett, A. Henderson (eds.), *Developing Learning Professionals*, Professional and Practice-based Learning 7, DOI 10.1007/978-90-481-3937-8_6,
© Springer Science+Business Media B.V. 2011

Beyond the mere articulation of these professional issues, it is necessary to assist students to develop strategies for personal coping. Workers in social and human services need to have a clear understanding of how they position themselves in the world of human service work because 'knowing yourself' is an important prerequisite to being an effective practitioner (Chenoweth & McAuliffe, 2005). This sense of self is a seemingly a mandatory prerequisite for effective practice and for being sustained as a practitioner. When effective strategies are developed, students reported feeling well-equipped to respond effectively to situations that they may encounter during practicums. An effective response through a comprehensive preparation can also assist them to facilitate the requisite changes for individuals, groups, and communities to whom they are meant to be providing a service. That is, beyond sustaining self, they are likely to perform more effectively in their important role.

The challenges discussed in this chapter are about the balance between ensuring that students are cognisant of the potential problems, yet are still motivated to engage and learn (i.e. they are not put off or disengaged by the prospect or actual occurrence of confronting behaviour). If this balance can be achieved, the students are likely to be well-equipped with a certain resilience that can lead them through their professional career beyond graduation. The danger is that, if not approached in a considered way, the preparation for the clinical practicum can create the opposite outcome. That is, students may feel inadequately prepared or unable to cope, which leads to withdrawal from the programme or, of even more concern, their development as ineffective human service practitioners. The focus of this chapter is, therefore, on using learning circles as a strategy for the development of human service practitioners so that they become secure motivated and capable practitioners who are able to deal with confronting situations that are central to productive and healthy professional life in human services.

The chapter comprises two sections. The first examines learning circles and the complexity of structures and processes used to ensure that the balance is obtained in the preparation of human services practitioners around confronting situations that can be unavoidable during their clinical practicum. These strategies are important for both the practitioners who prepare the students for the field and the students themselves. It is necessary for the purposes of effective practice to ensure that students remain in the field placement organisation to complete their programme even when they are faced with challenging situations; and further that they are not 'frightened' about going to placements where such situations might arise. The second section describes the outcomes of the use of learning circles as an innovative teaching tool to explore the dilemmas faced by students as they engage in lengthy practicum periods in organisations that support the well-being of individuals, groups, and communities. Further, this section examines the value of these circles as support for the students. A process for preparing students is subsequently developed from the discussion of the dilemmas and students' experiences.

6.1.1   The Balancing Act

As noted, a key challenge for the human services and social work curriculum is to find ways of preparing and supporting students for their practicums that will lead to students having a positive approach to engaging in their practicum, which includes preparing them for the potential of negative experiences, such as acts of domestic violence or neglect of children. The students may well encounter a range of traumatic situations whilst on their field placements. This is a difficult position as the teaching staffs do not want to 'scare' the students about the experiences that they may well have to confront. However, staff need to disabuse students of a 'romantic' notion of the role of a social worker or human services worker, that is the notion that those community members in need are easily directed and resources effortlessly sourced through the assistance of professionals, or that they will appreciate the efforts of social workers and human service workers, which can be particularly detrimental to the evolving sense of professional selves of students in this field.

Helpfully, university teaching staffs preparing students are often quite knowledgeable professionals from the field, as well as experienced in the delivery of field education programmes. These practitioners, because of their broad experience, are usually aware of the difficulties students may encounter in the field. These teachers are, therefore, mindful of providing a preparation programme that adequately equips students to identify the issues and work through a problem-solving approach to professional practice in a manner that is helpful to the community they are serving, and also protective of their sense of self. Inadequate preparation of the social work and human services workforce is believed to contribute to burnout (Lloyd, King, & Chenoweth, 2002). Individuals who experience high levels of emotional stress as they undertake their professional role, especially if feeling that they are not successful in helping clients, may begin to form negative sentiments about themselves and human service work. This can ultimately lead to poor work satisfaction and, eventually, may contribute to them leaving this form of employment. The intent, therefore, for preparatory programmes is to provide scaffolding to guide the novice practitioners who need to assist community members manage various difficult and, at times, tragic life circumstances. Such scaffolding is designed to ultimately prevent the burnout that can be experienced by professionals working in the human services sector, by preparing them adequately with strategies for dealing with this risk. The next section discusses the important role of scaffolding and its placement in the curriculum for preparing human service workers.

6.1.1.1   Scaffolding in the Curricula

Scaffolding refers to the manner in which university staff builds on students' existing knowledge and skills to enhance their learning. Scaffolding can be provided through the structuring of the clinical practicum within the curriculum. There are particular courses that include teaching activities and events that support the students' preparation and in-field education courses where targeted teaching strategies are used. One approach to this task trialled in an undergraduate programme is described as follows.

In the 1st year of the university programme, students are introduced to organisations and to individuals who contribute to the field placement programme in a session called Common Time. These sessions are designed to provide students with social and academic support within a flexible learning environment to assist their transition into university and their integration into their educational programmes and the field of human services. Students' skills and knowledge in areas such as essay writing, oral presentations, and professional development are enhanced through a mixture of structured academic and professional sessions which include contributions from guest speakers from the human service fields. Most importantly, Common Time provides the opportunity for students to establish peer networks and consult with teaching staff in an informal supportive environment. In the 2nd year of their programme, students undertake semester-long courses that provide them with more specific information about the roles and responsibilities of working in human service organisations. These courses are core elements of their programme and are titled and described as below:

- *Working in organisations* focuses on developing the skills and knowledge of students to work in human service organisations. Students will acquire an understanding of the organisational structures, accountability requirements, management responsibilities, and industrial issues which influence the nature of the work and work relations specifically in human service organisations.
- *Working in communities* introduces students to the theories and practices of community development within human service contexts. The evolution and current practice of community development are examined, as are the theories and key concepts underpinning practice models, strategies, and roles. Issues featuring in community work, such as urban planning, accommodation, and health are discussed with reference to particular community groups, for example women and families, indigenous and rural communities, and young people.

The exposure to human service and social work practice provided in these courses scaffolds development of the students' professional values and skills because they listen to the stories of successful human service and social work professionals. In the 3rd year of their programme, the students undertake an extended field placement (for the 3-year degree, this is their final activity). The students enrolled in the 4-year degree undertake a second extended placement in the final semester of their university programme. Together, and collectively, over the programme many opportunities for scaffolding that provide exposure to descriptions of confronting life circumstances are prioritised. These programmes support learners to understand and know about how to deal with the challenges as they are incrementally organised from awareness of issues, understanding the context in which these issues arise and how they might manifest themselves through to actual engagement in circumstances where they might encounter such issues. Because of its pertinence as a site in which these experiences may be first encountered, particular consideration needs to be given to the scaffolding for the field education component of the programme.

6.1.1.2 Scaffolding in the Field Education Component

In the human services and social work programme being referred to here, the field experience in community and government organisations comprises a significant educational experience that is intended to draw on and extend the educational experiences provided earlier in the programme. The duration of this field experience varies in length from 13 to 18 weeks. Four days of each week the students are in their field placement organisation. The 5th day is spent at university in classroom activities. This is a lengthy period to spend in an organisation especially when you are required to 'fit in' and demonstrate competence for dealing with confronting situations. The emotional toll of dealing with the challenges of the work on these novice practitioners can be detrimental if it is not carefully managed as it impacts negatively on their resilience and attitude towards the profession.

University staffs have structured this period into four phases – from orientation to exit from the organisation. The descriptions of the phases have a dual purpose. They describe the expectations of professional growth and development of the student and the task to be undertaken – see below.

Stage 1 – Orientation phase (off-site)

- The orientation phase involves an interview at the organisation and briefing sessions by university staff about expectations, procedures, and protocols.

Stage 2 – The beginning phase (on-site)

- The beginning phase occurs during weeks 1–2 of the placement. It is essentially a 'getting to know you' time and focuses on orientation and observation. Students should use this time to become familiar with the organisation staff, functions, and procedures.
- Assessment Task 1: During this period the students should be developing their goals in the learning plan in conjunction with their supervisor.

Stage 3 – The middle phase (on-site)

- The middle phase is the bulk of the placement where, as the student and supervisor feel ready, the supervisor will direct the student into an agreed and appropriate level of involvement, set tasks, and assignments. The student will be included in all decision-making pertaining to their areas of learning and responsibility. This is the largest part of the placement and the one that produces the greatest learning outcomes. Regular supervision time is essential here to monitor and assess the student's progress and capabilities. Students will be visited by their designated university supervisor and be required to participate in a three-way evaluation meeting with the university and field supervisors.

- Assessment Task 2: During this period students will write a weekly evaluation of their progress towards the goals they described in their learning plan.

Stage 4 – The final phase (on-site)

- Towards the end of the placement the student will be required to prepare for their departure. Students will finalise contact with clients or arrange handovers, finish administrative tasks and projects, and commence the processes of the final evaluation.
- Assessment Task 3: Students will complete their written assessment including a report about a special project undertaken whilst at the organisation and submit this to the field placement convenor.

However, despite the structuring of the field education period into these phases and the explicit statements about expectations for professional growth, the scaffolding was not sufficient to deal with the complexity of the emotional and cognitive development required by students to remain resilient when challenged by the confronting circumstances typical of daily work in the human services sector. If students were to be successful practitioners they needed to be encouraged to reflect about how they develop their self-identity as a professional. The dialogic of the reflective process encourages thinking about what has happened and how it can be changed.

Reflective practice is seen as a 'core activity' (Fook & Gardner, 2007; Moss & Petrie, 2002) for practitioners in the field of social service. It is understood as the ability to evaluate critical incidents within daily work and to use this evaluation as a means of improving practice and knowledge. This ability to reflect on practice has traditionally been offered as a way for practitioners to evaluate their own practice and the practice of others, with a view to developing their professional identity (Goodfellow, 1995; Mezirow, 1992; Patterson & Sumsion, 1996; Sumsion, 2003). Various methods of reflective practice are employed within the practice field, ranging from basic diary writing to the adoption of particular models, as a means of providing a framework for the reflective process. However, to reflect effectively, practitioners must see themselves not as the 'repository of objects of knowledge' (Moss & Petrie, 2002) but instead as creating new knowledge and understandings informed by contemporary theory, research, and practice. One way in which this process can be enacted and is aligned to the kinds of educational purposes being addressed here is through the use of learning circles.

Valuing the Learning Circles

Learning circles are sites of learning through shared inquiry and dialogue. The discussions start where people are at and involve a spiralling process of reflection and action. They were originally developed for American industries in the 1960s and later applied to adult learning for the purpose of promoting critical reflection amongst practitioners. A key feature of learning circles is that all participants are seen as being equal (Lovett & Gilmore, 2003). Sumsion (2003) states that the best principles of adult learning encourages and supports critical reflection about what individuals think they already know. Henceforth learning circles are a way for students to form new understandings with regard to important issues, in their own time (Gibson, 1998; Karasi & Segar, 2000). Learning circles are helpful in encouraging individuals to critically reflect on their values, attitudes, and practice with each other.

The use of learning circles in work-integrated learning programmes for the children's services sector has been proven to be a successful experience for helping practitioners, both novice and experienced, to understand and adjust to their chosen profession (Macfarlane & Cartmel, 2007). The practitioners in these programmes were aided in their ability to engage in professional conversations with colleagues. The programme arose out of the frustrations of university staff who are constantly involved in preparing mentors for students to work alongside in the children's services sector, yet who would then move on and are not available to mentor. The Australian children's services sector is under-professionalised and there is a high turnover of staff (Watson, 2006). Therefore, as one of the universities providing courses for this sector, there was a need to develop teaching approaches that would strengthen the professional links between novices and experienced practitioners, but at the same time not place further pressure on those working in children's services (Macfarlane & Cartmel, 2007). A teaching model called 'Circles of Change' was developed to be used within learning circles.

The intent of learning circles was to challenge thinking, that is to develop in students the ability to be critical and insightful thinkers. As critical thinkers they were able to reflect on everyday events and to consider changes to their practice. This process helped the students to make changes that would contribute to the well-being of the children with whom they worked. Therefore, the structure of the learning circles was extremely important. It was vital to use a model of critical reflection that would facilitate change in attitudes, thinking, and practice. The four-step model was in Circles of Change (Macfarlane & Cartmel, 2007). The first three steps – deconstruct, confront, and theorise (steps one to three) – teach students to inform their thinking through multiple perspectives in order that they might become more able to 'think otherwise' (step four) (Foucault, 1984) (see Table 6.1 – four-step action learning). This process enabled students to develop insights and explore ideas that would inform them around ways to deal with stressful situations (Macfarlane & Cartmel, 2007).

This Circles of Change approach also provided a process that enabled students and staff to understand the impact of the practices that were occurring in the field

Table 6.1 Four-step action learning model used in Circles of Change (Macfarlane & Cartmel, 2007)

Steps	Action
1. Deconstruct	Pull apart the main tenets of theory that govern particular practices and closely examine their make up, especially practices that have been enshrined as 'normal' and 'proper' practice. This stage is useful for prospective practitioners as a means of critiquing texts and understandings about practice
2. Confront	Approaching personal, social, and systemic issues head on by examining difficult, previously thought of as 'untouchable,' topics. This stage is useful for prospective practitioners as they focus on their own practice and confront issues that arise during the course of their day. The democracy and safety that Circle of Change provides and enables opportunities for more experienced practitioners to point out how important it is to confront issues pertinent to their own practice, for students to disclose any difficulties or uncertainties they may have and make the confronting process more understandable to the students engaging in it
3. Theorise	Carefully consider practice at all levels and question what is and what could be by thinking broadly. This stage is useful for prospective practitioners to understand the importance of linking theory to practice and the need to apply what is learned theoretically to what is implemented in the field. In Circle of Change students experience both academics and accomplished practitioners debating what constitutes best practice. They see the role theories and research play in shaping practice and identify what knowledge is privileged over other knowledge
4. Think otherwise	Challenge oneself to think outside the dominant frameworks and ideas and come up with other ways, or better ways of practising. This stage is useful for prospective practitioners as they recognise there are multiple perspectives and a variety of opinions about professional practice. As Circle of Change consists of experienced practitioners, academics, and students, and as each member contributes equally, then many perspectives are represented, explored, and contested

education settings. The university staff structured a teaching programme that had weekly learning circles as a core component. The reason for designing and enacting these learning circle tutorials in this way is to provide a 'safe' space for programme debriefing, to provide focused time to discuss workplace and practicum issues, to model critical thinking and reflection processes, and to encourage reciprocal and cooperative learning. The circles provided a safe place for these students and practitioners to consider professional practice (Macfarlane, Cartmel, & Maher, 2007). The learning circles were based on understandings and acknowledgement of the hard work of those who remain working in the sector. The privileging of time and space to converse in the learning circle did not place any additional burden on the workload of the practitioners. The workplace was not left with the sole responsibility of supporting the students. The university staff and the workplace supervisors worked in partnership to support the students.

In this way, similar parallels could be drawn between the children's services sector and the complexity of work in the human services and social work sector. The learning circle structure and process could be used to support the social work and human services students as they come to terms with confronting situations in their field education settings. The strategy has the potential to be adapted to the circumstances of large cohorts of human services and social work students engaged in extended periods of field placement.

Adapting the successful learning circle strategy used in the childcare field education required thoughtful consideration of the components of the process. In this case, the Circle of Change model (Macfarlane & Cartmel, 2007) provides participants with useful reflective tools and, as such, improves their capacity to engage in teamwork, collaborative decision-making, and reflective practices, and to finely tune generic skills required for effective lifelong learning and practice in the field. The model blends theoretical frameworks of community capacity building with critically reflective practices.

The reflective discussions allowed the students to consider their personal and professional attributes and their ability to use and develop these qualities as practitioners in social work and human services organisations. Initially, it is important that participants are accepted for their contribution and that recognition is given to the tacit knowledge (Cameron, 2000; Osmond & O'Connor, 2004) that each person already possesses. However, as discussions ensued in the learning circles, students created new understandings about their abilities to be effective in their professional role. Consequently, it was concluded that the learning circles were highly effective because the combination of the learning circle structure and the critical reflection process allows certain principles to be adopted. These include the following:

- An acknowledgement that quality is maintained through reflection on practice and through a focus on scholarship (deconstruct);
- The recognition that developing practitioners will face challenges in the workplace that may, at times, be overwhelming and that facing such challenges might require an examination of currents practices (confront);
- An understanding that changes in practice will only occur through engagement and dialogue with others and via an openness to the knowledge and expertise of others (theorise);
- A respect for individual and multiple perspectives (think otherwise);
- A focus on time efficiency and effectiveness.

These principles underpin development of teaching approaches that use learning circles. The complexity of the use of the learning circles is not to be underestimated when adapting the strategy to other circumstances. The context of the situation as well as the proposed content of the learning circle discussion needs to be managed thoughtfully.

Using the Learning Circles as Reflective Communities

The scaffolding of the curriculum and learning circles was a complex activity for the academic staff in their attempts to find the balance in activities required to successfully prepare human services and social work practitioners. It was further complicated by large numbers of students, and the length of the placement period.

In practice, academics were assigned to groups of 50–80 students enrolled in the field education courses. Therefore, for securing success with debriefing processes for students, it was important that they provided each other with support and not rely on the university academic. Further, it was essential that these gatherings of students in learning circles were held at regular stages (fortnightly) throughout the field education placement. Because of the nature of the field and the constraints and complexity of the work being undertaken it was important for practitioners to be continually reflecting on practice (Chenoweth & McAuliffe, 2005). The students needed to be able to help each other because the academic did not have the time to meet with each individual student to discuss their professional growth and the associated personal development. Consequently, this also modelled the potential for providing support for each other as practitioners once the students had commenced work in the sector.

In the learning-circles approach, the academics were conscious of teaching techniques for group reflection, as these were important to a successful debriefing process. The process relied on the students being able to support each other. Techniques for group participation, including ensuring each person spoke about their concerns, were critical to the process. The academic staff member moved between the groups of students listening to the conversations taking place. The intervention of the academic into the discussion was sometimes at the request of the students and at other times if the academic was aware of a 'teachable moment' they would intervene and question the student to confront the challenges they had identified or to highlight the potential challenges impacting on the student's practice.

During the orientation phase of the fieldwork programme, Stage 1, the students in the case described above were divided into groups which contained 6–12 participants who sat in a circle and partook in a four-step Circle of Change action learning model (see Table 6.1). Academics taught the students how to use the model to debrief about their field education experiences. They taught the students how to use learning circles within learning circles. To help initiate the discussion in the learning circle, the academic might suggest a focus to help concentrate the dialogue on a specific aspect of practice or the field education programme. During the orientation phase students were encouraged to consider the aspects of practicum about which they were most concerned as the focus of the discussion. As a stimulus to the learning circles, students were presented with examples of confronting circumstances that challenged the values and prior experiences of the novice practitioners. Prior to the shared discussion in the learning circle, students were asked to make individual written responses to the following questions:

1. What are you worried about as you go to placement (deconstruct)?
2. What will help you (confront)?
3. How will you go about this (theorise)?
4. How do you know that this has been successful (think otherwise)?

The students shared their written responses with each other. In the discussion that followed students were asked to consider things that concerned them (i.e. deconstruct), think about why they felt like that (i.e. confront), where they could source materials that would help them to resolve their feelings in order to practice in a positive manner for the people they were helping (i.e. theorise) and then describe what they would do differently (i.e. think otherwise). The written responses to the above questions formed a helpful basis for the data gathering process to gauge the effectiveness of the learning circle strategy. The students handed these responses into the academic staff who returned them to the students at the end of the placement period. The students re-read their written responses and made additional comments about the processes used to help them confront challenging circumstances.

During the initial weeks of practicum, in Stage 2, the students wrote their personal learning plan which contained personal and professional goals. This learning plan was important because it underpinned the professional development that students anticipated would occur during the placement period. The students were required to engage in reflecting on their professional growth through the writing of weekly journals. In the writing of their journal they were required to respond to four questions:

1. What progress has been made to your goal achievement (i.e. deconstruct)?
2. How have the macro-processes impacted on your goal achievement (i.e. confront)?
3. How does theory and literature help you understand your practice (i.e. theorise)?
4. What changes would you make (i.e. think otherwise)?

Students sometimes found it difficult to answer these questions in their journals if they have not had the chance to discuss their ideas with others. It is sharing with others that helped the students to consolidate their thinking about their experiences, because the consolidation though dialogue was a useful precursor for students before they wrote about their experiences. University staffs were aware that debriefing about the field experience was significant to the students' professional growth and competence. They provided opportunities for face-to-face debriefing in the form of fortnightly learning circles. The learning circles were planned as opportunities for the students to meet with their peers and university staff who were also challenged by similar experiences.

The links between the learning circles and the journal writing are multilayered. The learning circles are integral to fostering the language that enables students to express in written documentation their ideas about the practice in the field experience. The learning circles are facilitated reflective discussions that stimulate the students' thinking about their professional practice and provide the foundation for the journal writing. At the same time, the writing of the weekly journals provides the stimulus for the discussions in the fortnightly learning circles. Both strategies are linked to each other. Through the journal writing and the discussions of situations and potential feelings and responses students are assisted to explore personal coping strategies that will directly impact on the students' ability to deliver effective practice. These opportunities seek to find solutions for students for either practice with individuals or with groups and for their ability to deal with the complexity of the professional role they are undertaking.

The teaching techniques used by the academic staff require a synthesis of theory and practice. The learning circles are a rich source of conversation about practices, however, the dialogue needs to be shaped by the reflective questions in order to draw students' thinking towards possible solutions for coping with the confronting challenges. The synthesis is achieved using tools such as tacit knowledge, critical reflection, and mastery (Raelin, 2007). In the learning circles, the academics can engage the students in reflective conversations where the process of communication and language use is a form of 'knowledge production' (Raelin, 2007, p. 497). The students can articulate the multiple ways of thinking about the dilemmas they are facing. This thinking can be converted into actions and students are able to make choices from these actions to direct their practice. In turn, this concurrent reflection on experience will not only expand knowledge, but also improve practice. Raelin (2007, p. 498) states that it is 'through conversations with other local practitioners, and using detailed language specific to a function practitioners develop their understanding of how to engage with the task.' The learning circles are designed as reflective communities in which the students, through a dialogic process, learnt to reason together. Undertaking this activity fosters communities of practice that support a participatory structure that is inclusive of all students irrespective of background or field education experience. The learning circles allow the students to share their personal experiences about confronting experiences and their reactions. The students are able to discuss solutions to their emotional response and develop resilience to sustain their commitment to their human services and social work profession.

Successful Conversations

The learning circle strategy produced many successful reflective dialogues amongst students. In order to evaluate the effectiveness of the strategies the academic staff gathered students' perspectives in a number of formal and informal ways. The following section of the chapter examines the outcomes of the enactment of the aforementioned learning circles in a university setting. A key source of data was responses students made to the questions prior to going to practicum, during the practicum, and at the end of the placement period.

Over a 1-year period, the academics referred to above evaluated the learning circles intervention as a strategy for supporting students during field education. The staff collected data during the orientation phase as well as from the student journals and learning circles. Analysis of the data showed that the students found the learning-circle approach supported them during their placement. The learning circles were seen as a key educational intervention, because they provided the time and space for conversations that led to change in attitudes and practices, and were used here to prepare the students for the field placement experience. However, the main aim was for students to reflect upon their experiences in practicum settings and also share their learning with other students. The learning-circles approach was aimed to help them develop considered personal responses directed towards achieving the development of professional capacities and resilience that would be helpful during field education and when they joined the workforce.

The initial motivation for this project was a concern that human service students had reported being unprepared for the confronting situations they experienced in their practicums. Consequently, the learning circles concept had been introduced with a particular emphasis on preparing students for potentially confronting experiences through the development of resilience. Resilience here refers to the capacities to engage professionally and maintain a professional and personal sense of self in participation in human service work. As reported above, the learning-circles approach was used by students to be prepared for, discuss, and reflect upon issues which they found difficult or confronting. The students were able to exercise their rights to choose the focus of the discussions. The confronting experiences students reported were not only associated with the dealing with clients; they also referred to working with co-workers and supervisors who were not always supportive or considerate of the students' novice status. The students discussed many different issues and incidents.

Examination of the discussions in the learning circles and the documentation in the weekly journals found that the issues of concern extended beyond workplace issues to include personal circumstances. Students reported about the impact of their personal circumstances on their well-being and capacity to deal with the day-to-day experiences of the field placement experience. These circumstances had the potential to impact of individuals' ability to undertake their professional roles and responsibilities. Mastery of the management of personal circumstances gave the students confidence and agency to meet the professional demands of the workplaces. Simultaneously students' confidence and resilience were also evident in the manner in which they responded to workplace challenges.

The breadth of the students' concerns are evidenced in the students' responses contained in the transcripts from the learning circles and journal entries. These responses were able to alert the academic staff to the complexity of the issues that impacted on students' ability to be resilient in working with clients in vulnerable circumstances. The following examples are drawn from three student responses:

Example 1 – Leona

Leona was working with a client – a mother with a child with a disability who felt isolated and unsupported without any social networks. During the learning circle, Leona articulated the strategies she used to provide support for the client.

I helped a situation through my own personal experience. I relayed my personal experience and my coping strategies. I feel this lady realised someone does care about her. (Leona)

Leona's awareness of her professional skills including listening and networking were heightened as she shared her concerns with other students.

Example 2 – Rowena

Working with a client with mental health issues was a challenge that Rowena found confronting. She was distressed by the manner in which the client persisted in asking her if he could wear her glasses. Rowena discussed the context and circumstances with her student colleagues in the learning circle. She also described how she approached the client and she sought support for the approach she took.

The client pestered me for a turn to wear my glasses. I almost let him wear my glasses, as like my son, he was very manipulative. I was firm and told him not to ask again and that I would not let him wear my glasses. I wanted to stand by my boundaries. I realised that I could say 'no' to a client and I could say 'no' to my son, when he indulges in his manipulative behaviour. Doing this made me feel very empowered. (Rowena)

Rowena was able to test her ability to set parameters for relationships between clients and professionals within the environment of the field placement. At the same time, she believed that she could also manage her personal relationship with her son.

Example 3

Sarah was concerned about the negative and unprofessional behaviour of her workplace supervisor. She was uncertain about the potential consequences of her decision to confront the supervisor during her weekly supervision session. She discussed her concerns with her fellow students during the learning circle sessions. In discussing the kinds of strategies she could use to manage her situation, she decided that she would confront her supervisor. She used the learning circles to strategise about the process of confronting the supervisor.

I have been empowered for future practice particularly about using self reflection. I have also learnt how important it is to treat others with respect. (Sarah)

Sarah confronted the supervisor in a manner that had positive outcomes for the relationship between herself and the supervisor.

As well as the insight these examples provided for academic staff about the students' field education experiences, they also provide potentially valuable vignettes for use with subsequent student cohorts in the preparatory sessions. It is these kinds of experiences, responses, and reflections which provide an effective context for the students to consider how they will manage that placement and develop resilience.

The significance of critical reflection and collegiality was reinforced for the academic team involved in the project, as this opportunity had provided them with the platform for intense critical reflection on their work with students. Academic staff were forced to make the time to reflect on their teaching approaches and, further, they were alerted to the pressing issues that were concerning students. It raised awareness of the academic staff that they need to consider the experiences of the students beyond the often taken-for-granted assumptions about field education. Not only were the students engaging in processes of building resilience and agency to meet the demands of challenging workplaces, equally the university staffs were engaged in processes that provided insight and assessment of the effectiveness of their teaching approaches that would strengthen their capacity and agency to be effective in their role. The delicate balance between telling the students what they should do and leaving them to their own devices to manage their learning was a constant concern for the academics. Just as the students were dealing with vulnerable individual and groups, so too were the academics working with students often in vulnerable circumstances learning how to be effective practitioners.

Students identified professional capacities that they needed to develop if they were to be resilient to the confronting and challenging circumstances they would potentially encounter working in the human services sector. The professional capacities included:

- Self-reflection
- Empowerment
- Ability to say 'no' and not feel guilty
- Managing manipulative clients
- Ability to make a difference

The self-identification of the professional capacities required for the human services workforce is critical to professional roles and responsibilities of the sector as it works to achieve social justice, equity, and social inclusion. As mentioned at the beginning of the chapter, social work and human services are challenging. The personal context is a significant predictor of one's ability to be able to practice effectively as a professional in the sector.

Students also identified an additional range of coping strategies that were pertinent to maintaining their ability to successfully meet the demands of the field placement experience. These included strategies for managing the balance between work and personal life (e.g. don't take reading home, drawing boundaries, the importance of debriefing before getting into the car to drive home), methods for dealing with the realities of human service work and the differences between what is espoused in university courses and what transpires in practice (e.g. difference between ethics in practice and as taught at the university, practical and ethical issues, approaches to and concerns about contacting people unknown to you), and considerations for improving the educational provision (e.g. more preparation and debriefing for challenging situations, more preparation in interacting with clients and other professionals) as well as strategies that address the demands made by the practicum experience (e.g. balancing practicum experience with necessary paperwork). All of these are useful in supporting students' development and improving the provision both in university and practice settings. These strategies could constitute the basis of establishing a set of practices which might be useful for future students. Their evaluation particularly highlighted the importance of the preparation phase prior to the field education commencement. The academics have now introduced a field education preparation programme in the semester prior which contains a series of workshops on the topics identified as concerns for the students.

Further investigation of the students' data found mixed responses to the preparation process. Interestingly, some students reported that the concerns about confronting situation and the need to develop resilience had been overplayed and may have even caused unnecessary anxiety ahead of the practicum experience. Consequently, for these students some of the preparatory work seemed to be irrelevant because the reality had been far more benign than what had been predicted. Yet, university staff preparing novices for field placement and the workforce in the human services sector are constantly challenged to be mindful of the complexities that impact on the students' experiences in the field setting. The university staff came to be aware that there is not only one point in which they can intervene to support students to deal with confronting and challenging circumstances. Instead, the university programme needs an approach with multiple interventions that will support students throughout the field placement period to develop agency to most effectively integrate experiences in the practice settings with those provided through the university course.

The university staffs have revised the scaffolding of the curricula to include the following strategies and concepts:

Before the placement

Preparation for the placements includes opportunities to reflect upon and be advised about what is expected in placement. Staff discusses professional boundaries and how to maintain those when interacting with clients and other human service workers. Further they discuss strategies for leaving work behind at the end of the day (i.e. not taking the problems home with you); dealing with phone calls and difficult people; and developing resilience. Yet, within all this, there is not overt emphasis on the potential for confronting circumstances as, if overplayed, it might be generative of anxiety about practicum and professional practice more generally.

During the placement

Increased number of learning circles. These learning circles were extremely helpful because they included activities that were helpful for the students' capacity to manage their practicum experiences. The debriefing activities potentially will have a focus on personal as well as professional issues, for example consideration of debriefing processes, professional boundaries (i.e. their development and maintenance), and sharing and reflecting on challenging situations.

The staff uses the learning circles model for two distinct purposes. First, the learning circles are used as opportunities for students to reflect upon the totality of their experiences and share those experiences across the members of the learning circle. Second, the operation of the learning circle provides a model of ongoing professional development in which students can engage and which they can practice throughout their professional life. Debriefing about expectations, work requirements, professional practices, and capacities to work effectively manage difficult circumstances and leave problems at work are ongoing concerns as students move from novice to experienced practitioners.

The opportunities for 'real-world' experiences as provided in the field education for human services and social work students are significant to the preparation of effective practitioners. This is a highly complex activity for all involved. However, these opportunities need to be situated in a thoughtfully managed framework of curriculum and teaching strategies such as learning circles in order for students to maximise the professional learning from the confronting encounters. The learning circles need to be structured using a critical reflection model. Further, academics must be prepared to consider the impact of both professional and personal issues on students' capacity to develop their competencies as human services and social work practitioners. Consequently, academics and other professionals who are engaged in the process of practitioner preparation need to be prepared to use innovative and well-conceptualised strategies to meet such a challenge as well as ensure that their students do not become overwhelmed by what they might encounter in day-to-day operations.

Acknowledgement   The author wishes to acknowledge the support provided by the Australian Learning and Teaching Council for the inquiry referred to above.

References

Cameron, D. (2000). *Good to talk?*. London: Sage.

Cartmel, J., & Thomson, J. (2007). *Risky business*. Paper presentation at the Work Integrated Learning Symposium, Griffith University, Brisbane.

Chenoweth, L., & McAuliffe, D. (2005). *The road to social work and human service practice*. Melbourne, VIC: Thomson.

Fook, J., & Gardner, F. (2007). *Practising critical reflection: A resource handbook*. Maidenhead: Open University Press.

Foucault, M. (1984). Polemics, politics and problematisations. In P. Rabinow (Ed.), *Michel Foucault, ethics: Essential works of Foucault 1954–1984* (Vol. 1, pp. 111–119). London: Penguin.

Gibson, G. (1998). *A guide for local government on the theory and practice of learning circles*. Canberra, ACT: Australian Centre for Regional and Local Government Studies, University of Canberra.

Goodfellow, J. (1995). *A matter of professional style: Implications for the development of purposeful partnerships between cooperating teachers and student teachers*. Paper presented at the Practical Experience Professional Education Conference, Broadbeach, Queensland.

Karasi, M., & Segar, C. (2000). *Learning circles: An innovative tool for workplace learning for EL teachers*. Paper presented at 35th Southeast Asian Miniterial Education Organisation Region Language Centre Seminar, Singapore, 17–19 April.

Lloyd, C., King, R., & Chenoweth, L. (2002). Social work, stress and burnout: A review. *Journal of Mental Health, 11*(3), 255–266.

Lovett, S., & Gilmore, A. (2003). Teachers' learning journeys: The quality learning circle as a model of professional development. *School Effectiveness and School Improvement, 14*(2), 189–211.

Macfarlane, K., & Cartmel, J. (2007). *Report: Circles of change revisited*. Brisbane, QLD: Health and Community Services Workforce Council, Griffith University.

Macfarlane, K., Cartmel, J., & Maher, C. (2007). Circles of change: Innovative approaches to field education. *Every Child, 13*(2), 27.

Mezirow, J. (1992). *Transformative dimensions of adult learning*. San Francisco, CA: Jossey-Bass.

Moss, P., & Petrie, P. (2002). *From children's services to children's spaces: Public provision, children and childhood*. London: Routledge Falmer.

Osmond, J., & O'Connor, I. (2004). Formalizing the unformalized: Practitioners' communication of knowledge in practice. *British Journal of Social Work, 34*, 677–692.

Patterson, C., & Sumsion, J. (1996). *Linking theory and practice in early childhood teacher education*. Paper presented at the Australian Research in Early Childhood Education Symposium, University of Canberra.

Raelin, J. (2007). Toward an epistemology of practice. *Academy of Management Learning and Education, 6*(4), 495–519.

Sumsion, J. (2003). Rereading metaphors as cultural texts: A case study of early childhood teacher attrition. *The Australian Educational Researcher, 30*(3), 67–88.

Watson, L. (2006). *Pathways to a profession: Education and training in early childhood education and care*. Canberra, ACT: Department of Education, Employment and Workplace Relations.

Chapter 7
Reflective Learning Groups for Student Nurses

Jennifer M. Newton

7.1 The Need for Reflective Groups in Nurse Education

> ... as a student, I just feel like I'm just floating out there, I'm nowhere, I have no status I have nothing, ... I find it difficult other people controlling my life and I just stand there like a 3-year-old and have somebody watch me ... (Samantha)

Working as a competent nurse within a team of clinicians and alongside other healthcare professionals from other disciplines can be challenging for novice nurses. Recent research (McKenna & Newton, 2008; Newton & McKenna, 2007; Williams, Goode, Krsek, Bednash, & Lynn, 2007) reports new nursing graduates claim to be inadequately prepared for the clinical workplace and the associated responsibilities required as a practising nurse, including communicating and interacting with other and more experienced practitioners. Difficulties with assimilation are twofold. First, there is considered to be a mismatch between the experiences provided in the university setting and the practice setting. In particular, the pedagogical approaches currently employed in academia do not always adequately prepare graduates for the transition to their professional role. Second, while workplace learning support can be secured through the engagement of the learner with opportunities that arise and are offered through everyday work practices, new graduates often struggle with the reality of professional work (Boychuk Duchscher, 2009; Maben, Latter, & Macleod Clark, 2006). This shortcoming can be partially attributed to how as students they have been guided and supported through experiences in learning about nursing practice as they have transitioned to the workplace. This chapter discusses an approach to assist in the facilitation of student nurses' development of their professional role through the process of supported reflection. This is realised through the experiences of six students' participation in a reflective learning group during the final year of their undergraduate degree.

J.M. Newton (✉)
School of Nursing and Midwifery, Monash University, Melbourne, VIC, Australia
e-mail: jenny.newton@monash.edu

S. Billett, A. Henderson (eds.), *Developing Learning Professionals*, Professional and Practice-based Learning 7, DOI 10.1007/978-90-481-3937-8_7,
© Springer Science+Business Media B.V. 2011

The reflective learning group was offered as one strategy to assist students in contextualising their workplace learning and experiences in preparation for their impending professional role. Indeed, the reflective learning group was conceived to be an approach for clearing a pathway through the often impenetrable complexity of engaging in a healthcare workplace and contextualising and understanding the practice of nursing. Discussion also of how the reflective learning group supports the development of an agentic learner will be illustrated through appraisals of the students' learning and growth that emerged from their participation in this group.

7.2 From Ivory Tower to Swampy Lowlands

Schön (1983), in his seminal text on professional practice, describes the complexity of professional practice as one of murky lowlands that contrasts starkly with the technical rationality of what is taught in the echelons of academia. This, he suggests, creates difficulties for the practitioner when they graduate into practice. In professional practice, as in everyday life, our knowing is embedded in our action (Schön, 1983). Schön contends that professional education gives privileged status to systematic technical rational forms of knowledge and that there is a mismatch between forms of professional knowledge and the changing characteristics of practice settings which exist in any practice-based profession. The knowledge which professionals use in their practice is broad, deep, multifaceted and not easily articulated. In the swampy world of practice we need to refocus the problems in terms or contexts that can be understood by practitioners. This is particularly pertinent for learners as they juxtapose the parallel universes of academia and the organisational workplace.

There are many meanings attributed to reflection and how it should be utilised, and recent critique has challenged its inherent individualistic nature. Over the years, varying phases or stages have been identified that one can go through in the process of reflecting (Newton, 1999). For example, Mezirow (1990) sees the central function of reflection as validating what is known and, along with his associates, defines reflection as '... examination of the justification of one's beliefs, primarily to guide action and to reassess the efficacy of the strategies and procedures used in problem-solving' (p. xvi).

Mezirow (1990) makes the distinction between reflective action and non-reflective action, the latter of which entails both habitual action (e.g. driving a car or typing), and thoughtful action (e.g. playing chess). In thoughtful action, one is 'consciously drawing on what one knows to guide one's action' (p. 6). Habitual action 'takes place outside of focal awareness in what Polanyi (1967) refers to as tacit awareness' (Mezirow, 1991, p. 106). In contrast, reflective action, besides being a critical assessment of assumptions may, in Mezirow's view, be an essential part of decision making. Reflection can also be ex post facto, that is looking back on prior learning and the assumptions made on the content of the problem or the processes involved in solving the problem. This Mezirow (1990) refers to as critical reflection, through which new meanings and judgements can occur and this outcome he terms perspective transformation.

Recently Boud (2010) contends that reflection needs to be relocated in the context of practice, as in its current usage it often does not take into consideration the complexity of the workplace. Today's professional practice setting is changing and evolving; it has become collective in nature as opposed to individualistic, is multidisciplinary and there is an increasing emphasis on workers having to cooperate closely to enable each other to perform their job (Boud, 2010). He suggests that one should not lose sight of the original focus of reflection, which is constructing personal knowledge. Reflection 'is a means to engage in making sense of an experience in situations that are rich and complex ... ' (p. 29). Reflection thus can be considered an important source for practitioners to learn from their practice and come to a greater understanding of their workplace practices.

However, as a process, reflection is a cognitively demanding and complex skill that is not acquired overnight and requires carefully planned pedagogical strategies (Braine, 2009). Evidence suggests that students find it difficult to engage with tasks such as journaling or reflective writing if there is no assessment attached to them (Braine, 2009; Newton, 2004; Roberts, 2009). Reliance on students to journal, Burnard (2005) notes, can be problematic as many students collate piles of reflective accounts, a number of which could be fictitious. Indeed, Chirema (2007) suggests that while reflective journals are useful for promoting learning and reflection, they are neither the only nor the best way to facilitate student learning. This presents a challenge for educators in considering innovative approaches to assist students in developing reflective skills to maximise upon their learning opportunities.

7.3 Establishing a Reflective Learning Group

Numerous studies over the last decade have identified that some form of intervention is required to assist individuals to move beyond just a descriptive reflective account (Roberts, 2009). Given some of the inherent difficulties with reflection as an educator, I had previously drawn upon some alternate pedagogical approaches such as poetry, storytelling and creative arts (Newton & Plummer, 2009; Newton, 2004) that had been relatively successful. However, research undertaken with new graduates (McKenna & Newton, 2008; Newton & McKenna, 2009) suggested that engaging undergraduate students in a reflective group activity prior to the transition to the graduate year might assist in preparing students for their professional practice role, particularly as the current discourse on reflection suggests that provision of appropriate scaffolding and support is required to enable individuals to develop and engage in reflective practice (Roberts, 2009).

As part of a larger project exploring preparation for practice with healthcare professional students, a reflective learning group was piloted with a group of six 3rd-year undergraduate student nurses. The participants participated voluntarily following a presentation of the project to the 3rd-year undergraduate students during one of their key lectures. Initially eight students expressed an interest though only six actually committed to participation. The students were all female and ranged in age from 20 years to mid-40s. The students' engagement in the reflective learning group occurred for a variety of reasons, ranging from 'a fear of not feeling ready for the transition from student to registered nurse' to 'just wanting to understand a bit more about reflective practice.'

This reflective learning group was underpinned by the principles of action learning (McGill & Beaty, 2001). Action learning is designed to enable individuals to work with issues and to create action points that might be challenging but are focused and achievable. An action learning group can be facilitated by a member of the group or, as in this pilot project, by an 'external' facilitator that is not a peer. McGill and Beaty (2001, pp. 69–70) identify several core qualities that the facilitator should have. These include being real, genuine and congruent along with the ability to sense accurately the feelings and meanings a group member is experiencing and to convey this understanding to the group member. The skills of the facilitator are principal to the success of a student reflective learning group (Manning, Cronin, Monaghan, & Rawlings-Anderson, 2009).

In establishing the reflective learning group, ground rules were discussed and negotiated amongst the six students and were premised on confidentiality, honesty, providing constructive and supportive feedback, not interrupting, being non-judgmental and respectful, coming prepared and being committed to attend at least 80% of the planned sessions. This latter point is an important element of a reflective learning group (McGill & Beaty, 2001) to enable students to follow through with their action points. It is also important for the group dynamics to ensure there is some consistency in membership. The commitment to attend was diligently supported by the students in this group. McGill and Beaty (2001) suggest that to clear the mind an ice-breaker be used at the beginning of each learning group to enable the participant to focus their attention on being present in the group, and this was found to be a useful strategy in facilitating the learning group. On occasions, the ice-breaker activity actually triggered an issue that one of the students then presented. Students were also encouraged to consider journaling or writing anecdotes (see van Manen, 1999) to capture their experiences that they wanted to share and discuss. The students consented to the reflective learning group sessions being audio-taped and this provided rich data on the development of agentic learners and is presented in following section.

7.4 Forming an Identity

An important element of the reflective learning group was the expectation that the participants would identify their own action points at the end of each learning group and that these would be revisited next time they came. This was to encourage a sense of personal empowerment, and in doing so foster reflexivity and agency (Fook, 2010).

The ice-breaker activity frequently raised common trigger events in the reflective learning group that centred on the students' descriptions of a lack of affordances, that is not being provided with opportunities to engage in learning during their clinical placement experiences. These descriptions centred on a variety of negative feelings or thoughts, as illustrated in the words of Jess: 'I wasn't given enough freedom to practice ... I was there – I was allocated a preceptor [a registered nurse] for one day and I was sort of left at the sidelines, not really guided at all.'

Students described this type of occurrence as a barrier which prevented them from applying their procedural knowledge gained in the university to their actual practice in the workplace. Limited opportunities to engage were prevalent during clinical placements. Affordances in participative learning in the clinical workplace were constructed in a number of ways, illustrated in the following examples:

1. An increased power differential between student and professional nurse resulted in students' feeling inhibited, and this can ultimately lead to loss of personal autonomy. Students recounted experiences that created personal contradictions for them as they juxtaposed the role of a student while maintaining their individuality.

   > And they're marking you and you know you're going to have to be there and you want them to like you and all these other factors and it's hard to sort of take that sort of a, as an equal ... (Sally)

   > It's like you become a different person when you're out there as a student, you can be as, as assertive and authoritative as you want in your day-to-day life and then all of sudden you move into the student role where you just, ... like it's just so weird. (Donna)

   > like I was just a student and obviously not worthy of being there, um, um, and that I must have a long way to go still, when in fact I'm so close to being out, like just totally, you know, crushing your confidence. (Sheri)

2. Feeling burdensome reflected the students' dilemma of wanting to engage in learning opportunities but struggling with the belief that as students their presence generated more work for those supervising them.

   > Sometimes you feel like you're more of burden than a benefit to them (Jess)

   > He actually turned to me [referring to her preceptor] and said, don't interrupt and went back to work .... I think that that makes you as a student feel substandard (Samantha)

3. Being viewed as an outsider and transient; not part of the healthcare team. The students shared that they could not actively question practices they observed in the clinical workplace as they were very much on the periphery of the team.

   > You know, you don't really want to rock the boat (Sheri)

   > I guess it's just the whole rocking the boat thing and scared that one day I'll run into them again and I'm scared that they won't keep me confidential (Lyn)

   > Many of our issues are exactly that, they're about we don't know the boundary there and we don't know how to behave (Donna)

As these examples illustrate the experiences that were afforded to the students were clearly delineated. This prescriptive approach does not encourage students to explore and makes sense of the richness of experiences on offer that will ultimately assist in the development of professional knowledge integral to understanding the practice of nursing.

During the monthly reflective learning group the students dissected and interpreted the meanings of these trigger events. This developed through open facilitated discussion. Comparisons with standards thought to be expected by the profession and according to students' own clinical knowledge was a central focus of the discussions. The students shared their intuitive perceptions, often voiced through their own life and concepts of where the work event fitted in (as acceptable or unacceptable behaviour). Billett (2008) discusses how the learning experience of individuals is shaped by their earlier social experiences and that this pre-mediate experience shapes and construes the individual's learning in the workplace. Additional contributions of group members who recounted their own experience in similar situations enabled development of a perception of what was considered best practice (versus unacceptable). Lyn, for example struggled with nursing staff not taking enough time to communicate with patients, 'they don't seem to spend enough time with the patients, fully um, orientated, like on the clinicals while I'm doing something, I like to talk to the patients and then the preceptor sort of taps their foot behind you.' From her perspective Lyn had been taught that communicating with patients was an important skill to develop and sensed a dissonance with what she experienced in practice. Sheri, who acknowledged she set herself high standards, found the time issue annoying when learning to administer medications to patients, attempting to '... do the best and to make sure you don't make a mistake and my nurse working with me said "you're too slow you have to learn to trust yourself to a certain extent and speed up".' The reflective learning group provided a space in which the students could explore and challenge their values and assumptions about professional practice and organisational cultures and expectations.

Sharing such issues within the group broadened the students' perspective on engagement in and learning about workplace practices, enabling engagement and reflection about issues which they may or may not have personally experienced. The sharing of such professional behaviour issues fostered critical questioning by the students and in particular offered an opportunity for the more mature students in the group to draw upon their prior work life experiences and recount how they had managed difficult situations in other workplace settings. The resultant participative learning that emerged over the life of the reflective learning group engendered a changing perspective in the students' sense of identity as soon-to-be qualified professional practitioners.

7.5 Developing a New Perspective

Reflection on how learning opportunities are constructed and experienced by the students enabled some re-working of students' ideals with the groups' expectations.

Students' lack of confidence in the clinical workplace was a critical factor that underpinned the three main affordance issues alluded to earlier. Within most new learning situations, individuals' confidence can be reduced until they develop a degree familiarity within the workplace. However, in the case of the student nurses this lack of confidence during clinical placements negatively impacted on the students' communication with experienced nurses and members of the allied health team. A few of the students shared they were afraid in offering their opinion to other staff as their opinion might be wrong. This ideal was re-worked after realisation and confirmation by others in the group that, as third year students, they were not expected to 'know everything' and that it was permissible sometimes not to know. As Donna shared:

> Realising that I do know stuff, which I didn't think I did, I just think it's a confidence thing and having the support from the University is really important and a good preceptor. I think if I got, next placement I didn't get quite a, as a good preceptor, because I've have this wonderful start to this year, I'd be much more able to cope next time I think . . . .

Finding confidence was premised mainly in students' canonical and situational knowledge and centred on being given practice opportunities for self-development and then reflecting on these to gain greater insight into clinical situations. Through the sharing and drawing out of experiences, the students perceived a reduction in fearfulness of being regarded as not having adequate knowledge if they asked others for advice. The reflective learning group provided a pedagogical process to develop the students' capacity to be better prepared for facing problems and simultaneously working out how to resolve problems or issues at the time. Over the 7 months the confidence gained by the students enabled their skills and theoretical knowledge to be refined into understandings about actual nursing practices as they learned how nurses might behave in the workplace, enabling integration of these views into a personalised model of professional practice. Reflectivity became a tool for students to use as part of their repertoire of personal professional skills. In particular reflective learning was perceived as increasing the students' valuing of visualisation and giving them the skills and confidence to use in visualisation and critical reflectivity to reflect about a problem in its context, to resolve it and then be able to move on to something else. For example, how a new appreciation of the value of visualisation and self-talk as an adjunct to manage self-doubt and assist in confidence in the future is shared in the following statement.

> I want to really prepare for my next clinical because then that shows the nurses that we do have knowledge, and that you do have something maybe to give to the ward. And, just, in also increasing my confidence. Also to self-talk, like- I just say to myself: 'you know, I'm a good nurse . . .' (Sheri).

The students identified the need to develop a greater confidence in their everyday practice when on clinical placements in order to be perceived as final-year students and to achieve the identity of a 'professional nurse.' Lave and Wenger (1991) suggest that through participation in a social practice individuals form an identity associated with that practice. It would seem that some of this identity formation was enhanced through the students' opportunity of sharing practice experiences as they prepared for the transition to registered nurse. Indeed the students expressed that not only did the personal encouragement provided in the reflecting learning group help them find confidence, but also the discussions facilitated development of new perspectives about nursing practice.

7.6 Enhanced Professional Wisdom

Students perceived that involvement in the reflective learning group had a positive impact on their progression towards developing independent and competent nursing behaviours. This learning process was characterised by facilitative questioning and listening, which enabled the students to consider how it was possible to act more independently in the workplace through having increased insight into workplace culture and organisational demands.

> I think some of their [nurses] behaviour is there for a reason, like if is there a reason why the circle of nurses that we're getting preceptored by, is there a reason why they're behaving in a certain way, is it because of the acuity of the environment or is it a response to the way they've been educated or is it a response to the, an organisational response. (Donna)

Understanding how the organisational culture could influence the potential for learning to occur generated the following insight from Samantha, who was a mature-age student with prior experience as an enrolled nurse:

> ... if you have the preceptor who's prepared to let you grow, I think that's where it starts from, you've got to, as new nurses we have to encourage, and we have to change the way of thinking, and we have to be active in standing up for new nurses, because we cannot let the older nurses bully them. We need to say hey listen this is a new person let them go, give them a break because bullying is just crazy in nursing.

The students gained an awareness of how to create learning opportunities when working with their preceptor (an experienced nurse), as Lyn realised:

> I think it's okay to, tell the preceptor this is where I think I'm at and, and this is the level that I think I can perform to and then you know, that might be above what that preceptor thinks that I'm at, but they don't know me, so, but, if you tell them then, then they don't expect too little or too much.

Samantha also identified that she needed to 'be interested, ask my preceptor what do they want, and what do they expect from me,' and realised that she could secure greater affordances in her learning if she prepared 'the knowledge of where I'm going to [i.e., the clinical area], be good to myself, and I know that I do know stuff and know, that I am worthwhile and I can be assertive but nice.' A key focus in the development of agentic learners is the ability of the learner to actively and purposely engage in their learning in the workplace settings (Billett, 2008). With the support of her peers, Samantha was able to actively engage in her next clinical placement with renewed enthusiasm and purpose.

Over the period of the reflective learning group the development of the students' wisdom in dealing with interface of being a student and negotiating the boundaries of the workplace was exponential, and this was exceedingly encouraging for the facilitator. Fenwick (2008, p. 236) notes that learning is 'prompted by particular individuals, events, leaders or conditions. Individuals act as guides or mentors … leaders by encouraging inquiry and supporting improvisation and conditions by directing movement in particular ways … .' The reflective learning group in a sense became a 'community of practice' for these six 3rd-year students. Through the processes of shared meaning-making of ideas, subjectivities and practice experiences the students were able construct a sense of professional wisdom. This is exemplified in experience of Sally when she had a clinical placement on a palliative care unit and found herself providing care to a mother in her 40s, who was dying with cancer. Professional wisdom for this group of students encompassed learning the appropriateness of managing difficult, emotional practice situations. As a novice, with no prior experience of dealing with impending death, Sally raised the issue of dealing with emotions as a professional in such circumstances, as she found herself wanting to cry:

> I'm going to cry and I just had to turn away you know, like, it's hard because I just didn't know what to do with my emotions and I felt like it wasn't appropriate and like professional for sure, so I wanted to hide them …

Sally went onto to explain that the nurses,

> … were really old hats at it, you know, like I worked with a lovely nurse, for most of my shifts who gave a lot more, like stayed after and really was there for her patient, she gave so much more than just coming in and doing her work, but no, she wasn't like emotional, everyone knew it was sad …

The students shared their limited experiences of dealing with such emotional incidences in practice. Sally articulated that she had found this situation difficult. The group were challenged on whether it was appropriate to demonstrate emotion in front of a patient. Sally indicated that the palliative care nurses provided a little time to talk about this particular patient, during the nursing handover:

> We talked about it a little bit, but they [the nurses] weren't as like as I guess as raw as I am because, I haven't been exposed to it [dying] before and maybe my lack of life experience as well …

The collective and collaborative learning of the group in this instance resulted in a shared understanding of how to manage emotional challenging situations in professional practice. As the students gained greater confidence through their enhanced wisdom there was an increased willingness to be assertive and to proactively participate in the workplace when on clinical placements.

7.7 Identifying Learning

An evaluation of the reflective learning group was undertaken after 7 months. A colleague facilitated an audio-taped focus group interview with the student nurses to explore their learning. The interview was transcribed and thematic analysis undertaken. The central theme that emerged from the evaluation was that the learning group was of 'massive value.' The students shared that the reflective learning group offered more than 'the debrief' that is commonly offered by clinical educators when nursing students undertake clinical placements (Manning et al., 2009). The students gained a greater depth of thinking which helped their maturity as nurses and increased their confidence and reduced anxiety. The learning of new skills in relation to reflection saw the students shift from being esoteric to becoming more patient-focused in the context of nursing practice. As Sheri reported,

> ... I think it's just a growing experience, for me and building confidence and realising that I do know stuff, which I didn't think I did, I just think it's a confidence thing. I think it's given me identity. I feel like a nurse, whereas before I didn't when I went out.

Similarly for Samantha the reflective learning group gave her confidence and there was a transformation in her thinking '... this is not about me, it's about the big picture and I'm just a little girl in the big picture, it's put nursing and being a student into perspective, because I thought it was personal, but it's not.' Furthermore Samantha acknowledged that participation in the reflective learning group had assisted in her maturity as a nurse. Previously she reported that she did not understand what was going on, however, through the interactions with her peers '... now I see what everyone thinks, I know I'm okay now.'

7.8 Developing Agentic Learners

Supported reflection, which made use of group processes led by a skilled facilitator, was central to the students' development of their agency as learners. The reflective learning group allowed for consideration of multiple perspectives of practice issues not available to individuals engaging in personal reflection (Duffy, 2008). Within professional education literature Santoro and Allard (2008, p. 167) suggest that 'learning communities' are necessary for undergraduate students to develop reflective skills for future practice. The development of the students' agency through participation in this reflective learning group supports Boud's (2010) argument that reflection needs to be contextualised, embodied and co-produced; contextualised in terms of taking into account the actual people involved and the practice setting; embodied in the context of emotional engagement, that is participants must choose to undertake reflection and co-produced in that differences of power and position within the group are accommodated. The reflective learning group enabled students' values and understandings to be shared, debated, challenged and changed (Field, 2004). Moreover, the students articulated that the reflective learning group had given them 'a voice' and that they felt more prepared for professional practice as new graduates. Manning et al. (2009) similarly found that reflective learning groups provided undergraduate students with a sense of being valued and that their 'voice was heard.' The reflective learning group developed the students' agency, which is clearly illustrated by the following comment from Sally:

> The reflective learning group has taught me how to identify issues in my nursing and then address these issues, which has improved my nursing practice. I honestly believe that I have an advantage having participated in this research programme. I have learnt skills that I will use for the rest of my career and in my personal life.

Developing this group of 3rd-year students to become agentic learners was achieved through the promotion of collaborative learning, preparing them for the contestations they could encounter and encouraging critical perspectives on the students' experience of the workplace and the subsequent learning processes (Billett, 2009). The empowerment that being in this reflective learning group provided and the development of students' capacity as agentic learners was carried through into their graduate year programme as newly qualified nurses. The six individuals orchestrated their meetings and utilised this time to share and reflect on experiences of being graduates. This was despite some geographical hurdles of workplace locations across a city, and the realities of working full-time as health professionals enduring the competing demands of shift work and personal life.

As a pedagogical approach to enhance students' preparation before, during and after clinical workplace placements the reflective learning group provides, as the chapter has illustrated, an effective process to assist in the facilitation and development of agentic learners. While reflective learning groups can enhance the integration of workplace learning in the preparation for professional practice, it does require dedicated time commitment from both the learner and the educator.

Acknowledgements The author acknowledges the support of Robyn Cant, research assistant on this project, her colleague Lisa McKenna who facilitated the group's evaluation, the students who so willingly engaged and lastly Professor Stephen Billett whose Australian Learning and Teaching Council's Associate Fellowship (2008) supported this project.

References

Billett, S. (2008). Learning throughout working life: A relational interdependence between personal and social agency. *British Journal of Educational Studies, 56*(1), 39–58.

Billett, S. (2009). Realising the educational worth of integrating work experiences in higher Education. *Studies in Higher Education, 34*(7), 827–843.

Boud, D. (2010). Relocating reflection in the context of practice. In H. Bradbury, N. Frost, S. Kilminster, & M. Zukas (Eds.), *Beyond reflective practice* (pp. 25–36). London: Routledge.

Boychuk Duchscher, J. E. (2009). Transition shock: The initial stage of role adaptation for newly graduated Registered Nurses. *Journal of Advanced Nursing, 65*(5), 1–11.

Braine, M. E. (2009). Exploring new nurse teachers' perception and understanding of reflection: An exploratory study. *Nurse Education in Practice, 9*, 262–270.

Burnard, P. (2005). Reflections on reflection. *Nurse Education Today, 25*, 85–86.

Chirema, K. D. (2007). The use of reflective journals in the promotion of reflection and learning in post-registration nursing student. *Nurse Education Today, 27*, 192–202.

Duffy, A. (2008). Guided reflection: A discussion of the essential components. *British Journal of Nursing, 17*(5), 334–339.

Fenwick, T. (2008). Understanding relations of individual collective learning in work: A review of research. *Management Learning, 39*(3), 227–243.

Field, D. (2004). Moving from novice to expert – The value of learning in clinical practice: A literature review. *Nurse Education Today, 24*(7), 560–565.

Fook, J. (2010). Reworking the 'critical' in critical reflection. In H. Bradbury, N. Frost, S. Kilminster, & M. Zukas (Eds.), *Beyond reflective practice* (pp. 37–51). London: Routledge.

Lave, J., & Wenger, E. (1991). *Situated learning—Legitimate peripheral participation*. Cambridge: Cambridge University Press.

Maben, J., Latter, S., & Macleod Clark, J. (2006). The theory-practice gap: Impact of professional-bureaucratic work conflict on newly-qualified nurses. *Journal of Advanced Nursing, 55*(4), 467–477.

Manning, A., Cronin, P., Monaghan, A., & Rawlings-Anderson, K. (2009). Supporting students in practice: An exploration of reflective groups as a means of support. *Nurse Education in Practice, 9*(3), 176–183.

McGill, I., & Beaty, L. (2001). *Action learning* (2nd ed.). London: Kogan Page.

McKenna, L., & Newton, J. M. (2008). After the graduate year: A phemenological exploration of how new nurses develop their knowledge and skill over the first 18 months following graduation. *Australian Journal of Advanced Nursing, 25*(4), 9–15.

Mezirow, J. (1990). How critical reflection triggers transformative learning. In J. Mezirow & Associates (Eds.), *Fostering critical reflection in adulthood* (pp. 1–20). San Francisco: Jossey-Bass.

Mezirow, J. (1991). *Transformative dimensions of adult learning.* San Francisco: Jossey-Bass.

Newton, J. M. (1999). *Ways of knowing: Student nurses' perspectives.* Unpublished EdD. Melbourne, VIC: Monash University.

Newton, J. (2004). Learning to reflect: A journey. *Reflective Practice, 5*(2), 155–166.

Newton, J. M., & McKenna, L. (2007). The transitional journey through the graduate year: A focus group study. *International Journal of Nursing Studies, 44*(7), 1231–1237.

Newton, J. M., & McKenna, L. (2009). Uncovering knowing in practice during the graduate year: An exploratory study. *Contemporary Nurse, 31*(2), 153–162.

Newton, J. M., & Plummer, V. (2009). Using creativity to encourage reflection in undergraduate education. *Reflective Practice, 10*(1), 67–76.

Polanyi, M. (1967). *The Tacit Dimension.* New York: Anchor Books.

Roberts, A. (2009). Encouraging reflective practice in periods of professional workplace experience: The development of a conceptual model. *Reflective Practice, 10*(5), 633–644.

Santoro, N., & Allard, A. (2008). Scenarios as springboards for reflection on practice: Stimulating discussion. *Reflective Practice, 9*(2), 167–176.

Schön, D. A. (1983). *The reflective practitioner.* New York: Basics Books.

van Manen, M. (1999). The language of pedagogy and primacy of student experience. In J. Loughran (Ed.), *Researching teaching: Methodologies and practices for understanding pedagogy* (pp. 13–27). London: Falmer Press.

Williams, C. A., Goode, C. J., Krsek, C., Bednash, G. D., & Lynn, M. R. (2007). Postbaccalaureate nurse residency 1-year outcomes. *Journal of Nursing Administration, 37*(7–8), 357–365.

Chapter 8
Maximising the Integration of Medical and Nursing Students in Clinical Learning Environments: An Australian Perspective

Amanda Henderson and Heather Alexander

8.1 The Value of Interprofessional Learning

Effective teamwork in our complex and dynamic healthcare environments is essential to maximise patient safety and the coordination and best utilisation of the entire healthcare team. There is evidence that improved teamwork has a range of benefits. These include better workplace communication and improved coordination of service delivery, cost effectiveness, more holistic patient care, and more job satisfaction in the workplace through increased respect, understanding of roles and collaborative skills (Oandasan et al., 2006). Yet, although health professionals work in interprofessional teams immediately on graduation, curiously their education is almost universally within uni-professional courses. These courses likely provide limited opportunity for the development of collaborative teamwork skills in curricula or in assessment. Therefore, efforts to improve healthcare practice are increasingly turning to interprofessional education (IPE) as a means to develop skills essential to effective interprofessional, collaborative practice in health professional students.

Interprofessional education occurs when practitioners 'from two or more professions learn with, from and about each other to improve collaboration and the quality of patient care' (Barr, Koppel, Reeves, Hammick, & Freeth, 2005, p. xvii). This approach differs from multi-professional education, where different disciplines may share learning experiences (e.g., attending lectures together), but do not necessarily interact with each other, nor learn from each other, nor about each others' distinct practices. The Australian Commission on Safety and Quality in Healthcare (ACSQHC) (2008) has recognised that many critical incidents causing poor patient outcomes result from poor communication across different professional groups

A. Henderson (✉)
Queensland Health, Queensland, Australia; School of Nursing and Midwifery,
Griffith University, Queensland, Australia
e-mail: Amanda_Henderson@health.qld.gov.au

S. Billett, A. Henderson (eds.), *Developing Learning Professionals*, Professional
and Practice-based Learning 7, DOI 10.1007/978-90-481-3937-8_8,
© Springer Science+Business Media B.V. 2011

and different clinical settings. A consistent factor identified in recent international inquiries into healthcare systems where poor practices have been continued longer than acceptable is clinical settings where staff have not adequately communicated with each other, nor worked together effectively for the interests of their patients (Walshe & Offen, 2001).

Yet, there are also some cautions when advancing an agenda to improve communication across professional groups and clinical settings. Improving communication across and within teams can change the power distribution within teams, leading to tensions, and dilution of individual professional responsibility for clients (Colyer, 2008). Effective communication and collaboration can be hindered by personality clashes, professional territorialism, rotating team membership, and a culture of individualism. These potential problems necessitate that team members develop the skills and competencies to work effectively in interdisciplinary teams (Colyer, 2008). In this way, the development of highly functioning teams can be seen to be dependent on many factors, but particularly a culture of good interprofessional relationships of the members that comprise the team. It follows that interprofessional learning and practice are important considerations in the education of health professionals to develop these kinds of capacities. They can contribute towards effective communication and collaboration between health professionals and also across many professional groups to provide services that better address consumer needs.

This chapter discusses the importance of interprofessional education (IPE) as a foundation for effective teamwork. The emphasis, in particular, is on IPE as a work-integrated activity because such learning with other health professionals produces and enhances improved communication and integration of the members of the team. When IPE becomes embedded in practice, not only do students of all health disciplines interact to learn from and about each other, but also capacities (e.g., behaviours) commensurate with effective team work are developed. Such behaviours when modelled and practiced by clinicians can be instrumental in engaging students and, through collaborative practice activities, maximise learning opportunities. This outcome contributes to those professional behaviours that are 'learnt' becoming embedded in practice. In exploring IPE as a work-integrated activity, this chapter also identifies the many difficulties with the implementation of interprofessional education in the clinical context. Such learning is clearly important, though how this is best achieved is yet to be elaborated, because many of the studies available are small and context-specific, and do not offer general principles for progression. Investigations are limited in their broader applicability because the design of interventions is influenced by a range of factors, namely timing, availability of students, different curricula, diverse clinical settings, and the variety of health professionals and health contexts.

Nevertheless, this chapter offers a 'workable solution' that comprises a model of practice-based learning premised on a flexible and mostly self-directed interprofessional learning activity that can be undertaken in the clinical environment. This model is developed from a synthesis of existing accounts and a pilot programme undertaken by the authors. Although initially designed for medical and nursing students, this model could easily be applied to other professional groups. It is designed with the contribution of a facilitator to identify appropriate learning opportunities that can assist students and practitioners alike. Feedback from pilot studies of this facilitated activity indicates that students appreciate the opportunity to learn about each other's roles and to experience the opportunity to interact (Alexander & Henderson, 2010). This activity is based on the clinical environment and should be supported by a series of initiatives during the curriculum for developing students' interprofessional skills.

8.2 Aims of Interprofessional Education, Learning, and Practice

As noted above, the aims of interprofessional education, learning, and practice are broadly directed towards enhancing communication, collaboration, and teamwork to improve patient outcomes. More specifically, the goals of interprofessional education include the students' acquisition of the following knowledge, skills, and attitudes (amended from Barr et al., 2005), namely, students' ability to

- describe one's roles and responsibilities clearly to other professions;
- recognise and observe the constraints of one's role, responsibilities, and competence, yet perceive needs in a wider framework;
- recognise and respect the roles, responsibilities, and competence of other professions in relation to one's own;
- work with other professions to effect change and resolve conflict in the provision of care and treatment;
- work with others to assess, plan, provide, and review care for individual patients;
- tolerate differences, misunderstandings, and shortcomings in other professions;
- facilitate interprofessional case conferences, team meetings, etc.; and
- enter into interdependent relationships with other professions.

From this listing, it can be seen that the educational purposes here are about understanding individuals' own and other forms of professional practice, the parameters of the use of these practices, the scope and limitations for collaborative practices, and the kinds of capacities required for effective interprofessional work. For these competences to be achieved, educational practices need to be aimed at the following: (i) addressing negative professional perceptions; (ii) deepening insights into each other's roles; (iii) enhancing interprofessional communication; and (iv) preparing students for interprofessional work (Reeves & Freeth, 2002). Together, these purposes elaborate the bases for realising an effective interprofessional educational provision. However, before discussing provisions for interprofessional learning, it is important to understand the kinds of impetuses that have led to demands worldwide for improved interprofessional education, learning, and practice.

8.3 The Impetus for Interprofessional Education

The impetuses for interprofessional education are long-standing, powerful, and growing in emphasis and scope. Political agendas and local unit cultures have had a major impact on the imperatives for interprofessional development in the curricula of health disciplines designed to promote interaction, education, learning, and practice across areas of professional practice (Barr, 2002). These impetuses have led to interprofessional education and learning being introduced internationally, albeit with varying levels of commitment and uptake, in an attempt to improve the quality healthcare provision issues identified as requiring this initiative.

At the pedagogic level, interprofessional education has been sporadically attempted through a range of teaching activities such as problem solving, small group work, clinical activities, and attendance at common lectures. Internationally, the effectiveness of interprofessional education is beginning to be established from preliminary evaluations of these teaching and learning strategies. In particular, favourable outcomes are emerging around the areas of improving attitudes towards members of other healthcare disciplines, increased knowledge of each other's roles, and enhancing teamwork. This work is further fuelling energy and commitment in this area with national agencies being established in many countries to promote the healthcare workforce (e.g., Health Workforce Australia). Although receiving considerable attention overseas, there has been little discussion or debate around the merits of IPE in Australia until relatively recently (Stone, 2007). The importance of enabling systems that foster interprofessional teaching, learning, and practice are now being recognised at the national level in Australia. In particular, the recognition that teamwork can address many issues pertaining to safety and quality has assisted the momentum of IPE. The National Patient Safety Education Framework (ACSQHC, 2005) provides curriculum guidelines that build teams and collaborative working relationships so that enhanced patient safety can be achieved.

In the first instance, a key concern is the limited emphasis on teamwork and building relationships in curricula of the health disciplines. The National Patient Safety Education framework identifies that health professionals need to know who is on their team, understand roles and characteristics of teams, realise the importance of establishing clear goals and objectives, and, therein, understand why team functioning is important for healthcare quality, including the reduction of errors (ACSQHC, 2005). The structure of curriculum for health professionals across Australian universities generally does not provide for this sequential learning about team functioning while at university, nor through associated relevant experiencing of team work that would be expected during clinical practice. In particular, the clinical practice experience across all health professional groups is focused on the development of profession-specific knowledge (Hall & Weaver, 2001). The challenge for health professional education is to introduce communication and teamwork in a meaningful manner so students recognise the relevance of such learning.

8.4 The Potential Positive Impact of Interprofessional Education

The potential of IPE is held to be significant, as can be seen from the case made above. Yet, to appraise that potential, it is necessary to understand something of its worth: its latent positive impact on healthcare practice. Potentially, interprofessional education can improve organisational practice and staff satisfaction. Examples of this are evident through teams working together on 'simulated cases.' Groups of health professionals who normally work together in a specialised sphere of practice, for example, student midwives, doctors and nurses (Furber et al., 2004); palliative care staff (Wee et al., 2001); community health nurses and social work students (Russell & Hymans, 1999); medical students participating in emergency training with paramedic students (Hallikainen, Väisänen, Rosenberg, Silfvast, & Niemi-Murola, 2007); and mental health practitioners across a range of health disciplines (Reeves, 2001) have positively evaluated opportunities to learn and work together. Positive changes in students' understanding and cooperation during planned and facilitated interdisciplinary experiences have also been verified in specialised settings, such as aged-care mobile service delivery (Hayward, Kochniuk, Powell, & Peterson, 2005), and rural and remote settings (Dalton et al., 2003; McNair, Brown, Stone, & Sims, 2001).

Thus far, in Australia, most work has been initiated locally, within a school, or across a couple of schools at a university, and in collaboration with a number of health-service districts. These programmes have been most successful in rural and remote communities (McNair et al., 2001), possibly because of the need for and practice of interprofessional learning in these settings. A programme designed to expose medical students to the work of health professionals during a community placement has been evaluated as successful in medical students obtaining relevant clinical skills for use upon graduation (Young, Baker, Waller, Hodgson, & Moor, 2007). Yet, it remains uncertain whether these kinds of experiences make a difference to how medical students interact with other health professionals. Except for these small-scale initiatives to facilitate work practice between medical, nursing and allied health profession students predominantly in rural and remote areas, there has been little systematic effort in Australia to foster interprofessional education at the undergraduate area in the acute clinical context.

As identified by Reeves (2001), the value of sustained outcomes from many of these studies is still uncertain. Positive changes to organisational practice from these activities are fairly weak in justifying changes over a longer time frame. While short-term benefits are evident in the literature, there is an assumption that the practice changes that result from these one-off endeavours are embedded within team functioning. The challenge for IPE to be effective in the longer term is to ensure that communication and collaboration in clinical practice situations are sustainable and continue beyond these single interventions. If these behaviours are continued and, therefore, role modelled, they are more likely to be adopted and incorporated into the practice of the students who experience their clinical practicum in these areas. The need to establish the relevance of collaborative activities is not confined to learning and teaching in the university curricula but extends to early clinical practice experiences in the undergraduate curriculum. If practices observed by students from the outset of their clinical experience are demonstrated to result in effective working relationships across professional groups, then interprofessional learning is more likely to be sustained (Pollard, 2009).

8.5 Interprofessional Learning in Clinical Practice-Based Contexts

A key issue for effective interprofessional practice is its introduction at the undergraduate level. The majority of the research has been conducted with health professionals after registration (i.e., with existing teams) and, therefore, at the completion of their degree studies. There is a strong argument suggesting that interprofessional activities should be introduced early into undergraduate programmes so that students in these professions become familiar with this concept and its practices from the commencement of their studies. Further to this, interprofessional practice needs to become evident within clinical practice settings both through the observation of interprofessional practice between clinicians and engagement of students across different health discipline groups. Making this opportunity available is essential both as a strategy for allowing students to observe interprofessional work and also for them to engage in and develop the capacities for that kind of work.

However, these initiatives are ambitious, because of existing professional and institutional barriers. The reality of putting into operation learning arrangements of this nature, particularly in clinical settings, is complex and full of challenges. In many clinical settings, communication and collaboration across professional groups, precursors of interprofessional practice, are often not obvious to students situated in the practice environment (Ross & Southgate, 2000). Furthermore, there are many impediments to bringing students of the different health disciplines together. Medical and nursing curricula are conceptually very distinct with medicine increasingly a graduate entry course. Although often offered as a graduate entry course, nursing education is mostly undertaken through undergraduate courses. Attempting to facilitate integration across professional groups (e.g., undergraduate nursing students working with postgraduate medical students) is fraught with logistical difficulties. These difficulties are not necessarily a result of attempts to meet educational needs, but rather traditional patterns of teaching unique to each profession.

In many of the curricula within the health professions, even when students are learning common skills and content, they usually do so without interaction with students in other health professional programmes (Barnsteiner, Disch, Hall, Mayer, & Moore, 2007). This is because these educational provisions have until now been organised quite separately, and have distinct entry requirements, programme structures, and content. There is also a lack of collaborative history and links between and within universities in issues associated with promoting interprofessional work within clinical settings (McNair et al., 2001). Shared learning is neither practiced nor valued across many medical and nursing curricula (Barnsteiner et al., 2007).

Because of its recent introduction, obviously, the vast majority of current health professionals did not train in an interprofessional environment and many do not practice in such and, therefore, are not in a position to create such learning opportunities for students during the clinical practicum experience (Curran, Sharpe, & Forristall, 2007).

These historically derived discipline-based differences are evident in curriculum, planning aspects, and assessment approaches of health professional programmes. They comprise issues associated with numbers, availability, and academic ability of students. In many faculties of health sciences where medicine and nursing students are likely to be enrolled, the number of students for these tertiary programmes can also differ markedly, making pairing kind of arrangements impractical. Schools of nursing in more recent times have been increasing numbers to ensure an adequate number of professionals in the skilled workforce. While medicine has also been under similar pressure, the numbers required are generally not as high as within nursing. This inequity of numbers results in the greater availability of nursing students than medical students during clinical practicums, which can restrict the opportunities for interprofessional student engagements, such as pairing or joint clinical placements. A further complication is the different academic levels between students that require consideration when partnering them during clinical placements (Dalton et al., 2003). Consequently, the selection of students to participate in interprofessional learning activities needs to take account of balancing students according to the year of study or comparable training level (Anderson, Manek, & Davidson, 2006). All of these matters are not easily reconciled.

There are also issues associated with the supervision arrangements within the actual clinical settings. These quite distinct and different arrangements for students make the logistics of engagement in an interprofessional activity even more difficult. Students are placed throughout the hospital attached to their uni-professional placement coordinator and integrated within their respective professional groups each with a distinct modus operandi (Anderson et al., 2006). While both nursing and medical students are supernumerary and mentored by a range of frontline professionals (Anderson et al., 2006), medical students are attached to a medical team that conducts their professional practice based on the geographical location of their patients. This may be confined to one ward or may be across a number of wards or units and in outpatient departments. Alternatively, nursing students are usually placed in a single geographical unit where they learn the routines established around caring for patients. Indeed, these kinds of models of nurse education are increasing as there is seen to be value in student nurses returning to a clinical environment with which they are familiar and in which they can engage more effectively (Henderson, Twentyman, Heel, & Lloyd, 2006).

In addition, there are other orthodoxies which work against easy integration of interprofessional preparation. These include the different disciplines each having distinct understandings of teamwork; that is, nurses describe collaboration as having input into decision making while physicians describe it as having their needs anticipated and directions followed (Makary et al., 2006 cited in Barnsteiner et al., 2007). This lack of alignment may contribute to students' perception that there is little to be achieved through involvement in interprofessional collaboration. Furthermore, participation in these activities is often not assessed or carries minimal weighting (Anderson et al., 2006). Assessment is, instead, focused on profession-specific skills. Medical students, in particular, have been identified as being reluctant to participate in interprofessional working and learning as they do not see development of teamwork as relevant to professional ability (Reeves & Freeth, 2002). Given what has been discussed above, this response is perhaps not surprising.

Clinical learning is also time-pressured given the requirements for content-specific knowledge to be 'learnt' during the practicum in which clinical activities need to be performed. This lack of time is yet another barrier to informing and changing attitudes needed for effective interprofessional learning and practice (Steinart, 2005). Health practices, including traditional hierarchies, work against the easy introduction of interprofessional work and interprofessional education. This situation is, in part, contributed to by practices within educational institutions whose orthodoxies work against, rather than for, more collaborative forms of working and learning across the professions. Consequently, to advance the prospects for promoting interprofessional practice, and for acting and educating interprofessionally, there are a range of factors which must be addressed to embed interprofessional learning within clinical settings. The success of any activity is most probably derived from the learning opportunities that students perceive arise from the experience. We identified that success was more likely if we presented students with a unique learning opportunity than if we broke down barriers.

8.6 Considerations for Designing Practice-Based Interprofessional Activities

In considering how interprofessional activities might best progress, arrangements that focus on core concerns for healthcare practice may provide a better opportunity than attempts to reorganise long-standing healthcare work and institutional practices. The logistics of conducting collaborative clinical activities across disciplines stand as major barriers to the conduct of interprofessional education in practice settings (Barker, Bosco, & Oandasan, 2005). As discussed above, education structures and healthcare institution arrangements continue to silo the professional groups. When exploring how best to develop a clinical activity that bridges health professions, in this case, medicine and nursing (Alexander & Henderson, 2010), we found it worthwhile to focus on the care of the patient. These professions routinely come together to address the patients' needs and, therefore, focusing on the patient was seen as worthwhile to assist in addressing the identified barriers. When the patient is identified as the priority, then learning through interactions with the patient and the medical and nursing students is based on the knowledge and prior experiences of the patient, and of the nursing and medical students. This activity places patients as the basis of interactions between medical and nursing students.

Table 8.1 Addressing logistical issues in the clinical setting

Barriers identified in the literature	Design considerations needed to address barriers
Numbers of students in different professions	Activity needs to be flexible and students able to pair up according to availability (if fewer medical students than nursing students – medical students participate more often).
Availability of students (time, rostering)	Actual participation in activity needs to be jointly negotiated by students, clinical preceptors, and local staff. Activity also needs to be flexible to overcome the difficulties with timing and rostering.
Different year levels, academic ability, maturity of students	Activity needs to be designed so that learning focuses on generic content and process issues, e.g. roles/responsibilities, rather than content issues. Process issues are not delineated on year levels and academic ability. This also allows students to investigate discipline-specific issues and needs.
Different supervision arrangements	A generic facilitator is needed to locate and match student pairs in geographical locations that overcome the differences in supervision arrangements.
Health education takes place in a silo	The activity needs to be engage students in a key situation where the silos are not separate.
University curriculum and assessment structures, scheduling	A common clinical placement time needs to be identified; the activity needs to be short and able to be repeated on multiple occasions.
Tension between profession-specific tasks and time for IPE	The activity needs to be designed to augment discipline-specific tasks and be flexible so it can easily accommodate attendance at other required commitments.
Space	Early organisation of room space for meetings with the facilitator.
Facilitator time/Workload pressures	Activities need to be facilitated through extra clinical support.
Ethos of clinical area	The activities needs to be supported through the leadership team and reinforced through local ward practices so that they become meaningful to the students.

Our study found that students can meaningfully interact when collaborating on patient care. Using patient care as a basis, Table 8.1 identifies the barriers to IPE identified in the literature and describes specific interventions that should be included in the design of the interprofessional learning activities. In the left column of this table are the issues identified in the sections above that represent barriers to effective enactment of interprofessional practice and, consequently, its learning by healthcare students. In the right column are potential responses to these barriers.

The development of the components of the interprofessional learning activities identified above needs to be carefully considered and planned for to facilitate their effective enactment in clinical settings. This enactment is important because interprofessional learning and teaching activities often do not explain the detailed procedural components that ultimately lead to the success or demise of the activity. For example, Freeth, Hammick, Reeves, Barr, and Koppel (2005, p. 54) identify that 'studies do not convincingly demonstrate cause and effect [so] there remains a problem in justifying the value of interprofessional learning.' The following elaborates a flexible activity that can be undertaken by medical and nursing students in the clinical setting to redress this kind of barrier.

8.7 An Interprofessional Clinical-Based Learning Activity for Medical and Nursing Students

The value of this activity is that it is patient-focused and designed to be used flexibly in busy clinical environments. It involves pairing just one medical student with one nursing student in a self-directed, structured activity, designed to enhance learning through collaborative engagement of the students with a facilitator on completion of the activity. Ideally, the activity is conducted in a sequential manner but can also be interrupted if necessary by service demands or teaching activities. Discussion with a facilitator is an important component of the activity because the facilitator can guide the learning and reflection that arises from interprofessional engagement. In addition, a workbook guides the discussion between the patient and the students. The workbook is not a 'written exercise' that focuses students in an isolated documentation activity. Instead, the workbook through broad questions assists the students engage in dialogue with the patient and with each other. Moreover, it specifies the following steps for the students to perform:

- Step 1: The students familiarise themselves with the patient notes, in particular, the reason for admission and complete Section 8.1. In Section 8.1, the students are asked to note the patient's age and gender; and then summarise the patient's medical history from the admission notes. From the notes, the students derive the present health complaint of the patient.
- Step 2: The students interview the patient together, using Section 8.2 of the workbook as a guide. Each student completes an individual workbook. In Section 8.2, students are asked to explore with the patient their understanding of their reason for admission, and what they expect will happen. Patients are also asked about their social situation, and to identify everyone who contributes to their care.
- Step 3: The students work through Section 8.3 of the workbook together. This section asks the students to prioritise the patient's problem list, namely, to list the staff involved in the patient's journey and to identify barriers to the patient's progress. They are also asked to describe, compare, and contrast each of their health professional roles in the care of the patient. They are also asked to consider patient safety issues.

- Step 4: The students discuss their experience with an IPE clinical facilitator. This discussion is guided by a series of structured questions provided to the facilitator who explores differing perceptions of care, patient safety issues, and what students learnt about each other's roles.

Through this kind of activity, students engage in an interactive exercise focused on developing communication and understanding of others' roles that can be readily repeated. It is quite different from other approaches to interprofessional learning where students take on workloads in teams. The advantages of this approach are that it is relatively easy to organise and is of a scale that is realisable, because it is the students rather than the healthcare system that undertake the organisation and progression. Through engagement with the activity students can subsequently initiate further interprofessional activities. There is potential for this to occur where interactions that rely on collaboration across health professional groups are routinely embedded in healthcare delivery.

8.8 Sustainability: Key Factors for Embedding Interprofessional Learning Activities

Medical and nursing professionals serve as strong role models for students during the clinical practicum and, therefore, are in a powerful position to influence attitudes and behaviours towards interprofessional learning. However, many of these professionals have not practiced, and do not practice, interprofessional work. Therefore, they are not well placed to encourage, support, and sustain these practices. It follows that strategies need to be developed and intentionally enacted within clinical settings to influence and enable interprofessional student learning. From an analysis of the available literature, it is possible to identify three key factors that are needed in the clinical contexts for interprofessional learning to be observed and activities such as just described facilitated within the clinical context: (i) leadership, (ii) involvement of clinicians, and (iii) relevant clinical activities. These factors are now briefly discussed.

8.8.1 Leadership

Leadership is a key issue for IPE (Steinart, 2005). Senior leader support is essential, otherwise the practice will not occur (Barker et al., 2005). Leadership support is not merely the acceptance of the activity but rather role modelling interactions. Clinicians need to be champions of interprofessional learning and work (Ross & Southgate, 2000). The types of activities that could be championed by clinicians include medical and nursing discussions during ward rounds, however, often 'rounds' are performed without a representative from the nursing staff. Doctors will write messages in the chart to communicate to the nursing and allied health staff:

Table 8.2 Recommendations for engaging leaders through the continuum

Leadership support	Suggested actions
Senior management – for access and permission to approach middle management about the project.	Liaise with the following staff: Health-service medical and nursing executive group Nurse educators Nursing clinical coordinators University School of Nursing University/health-service joint clinical placement coordination committees University School of Medicine
Local management – continuous presence to remind and reaffirm the staff who are able to directly influence the participants of the project	Enhance support through Personal introduction to all local nurse unit managers, team leaders, and many of the staff on the shift where and when the nursing and medical students work. Reinforcement through the employment of facilitators to introduce themselves. Conduct numerous information sessions with clinical staff; in particular, identify the most strategic meetings, and provide regular short sharp information.

However, students do not observe health professional interactions. These local practices are pivotal in the messages they communicate to students. In promoting IPE, it is imperative that all levels of clinicians (including senior management) are aware and supportive of the activity to be conducted. Extensive liaison and consultation needs to be undertaken with staff within the clinical context. From experience, while the hospital executive staff can be keen to progress interprofessional activity, 'buy-in' is needed by the middle levels of leadership within local contexts (i.e., those with leadership roles in particular wards or clinics). Therefore, it is recommended that 'buy-in' is sought through presentations, meetings, and workshops. These kinds of forums are needed to inform and educate key staff, from those at senior executive levels to staff at the bedside, in clinical contexts where students are located. The types of presentations and meetings are listed in Table 8.2.

8.8.2 Clinician Involvement

As student learning during clinical practice is largely through the observation of and the practice of interprofessional learning, then interprofessional activities need to be demonstrated through regular ward behaviours, and students need to be facilitated to engage in learning exercises, such as the activity outlined earlier. It is essential that clinicians are treated as a strategic component of IPE because highly skilled clinicians are needed to support and guide student learning through interprofessional activities (Freeth et al., 2005). Moreover, clinicians need to act as local champions in communicating and convincing both staff and students about the benefits of interprofessional learning (Baker et al., 2005). These local champions can also contribute to organisational ownership (McNair et al., 2001). It follows then that clinicians who already practice behaviours commensurate with interprofessional education need to be engaged (Curran et al., 2007). However, it is acknowledged that without the leadership described above, this practice may be very limited in its success.

As previously explained, clinician involvement is difficult to secure. Clinical staff with their own workload rarely have time to support the student in interprofessional activities, therefore co-support of a university clinical facilitator can assist the student reflect (Freeth et al., 2005, p. 104). The use of non-discipline-specific clinical facilitators is often crucial in the initial engagement of students to participate in IPE activities until clinician involvement is confidently secured (Oandasan & Reeves, 2005). The role of these facilitators is diverse, but includes: (i) having contact with staff and students; (ii) development of an active learning environment; (iii) development of student capability; (iv) mentorship; (v) conducting tutorials; (vi) support groups; and (vii) liaison with management. It is recognised that there is capacity for all clinicians who are employed as a 'clinician teacher' or placement supervisor to be able to foster learning across all discipline groups (Emerson, 2004). Yet, at this time, the literature offers little in empirical approaches to enhancing the effectiveness of a facilitator. This circumstance, however, is consistent across all the health professions. There is considerable descriptive work but little empirical findings about the value of facilitators and how they work of the kind that will be acceptable in clinical practice. In particular, such facilitators need good group-work skills.

There are often tensions in the relationship of the facilitators with disciplines that are not their own (Thomas, Clarke, Pollard, & Miers, 2007). Facilitators can find it difficult to simultaneously promote discipline-specific knowledge, and also the skills of teamwork and collaborative practice. While there is little evidence about the efficacy of work of facilitators, those facilitators who promote collaboration in an attempt to foster IPE do suffer from 'burn out' as the work involved in drawing the teams together to support student learning is immense and intense (Reeves & Freeth, 2002). This observation may be indicative of the confidence that they have in the environment where they are employed to facilitate. Success is related to the experience and skill of facilitators more than to a precise method used (Barr, 2002).

A clinical facilitator can assist with those immediate issues, such as timing, where students prioritise a profession-specific task and cannot identify how they will commence an IPE activity. In situations such as this, facilitators can assist students build the activity in a flexible fashion and, furthermore, assist clinicians and students to identify that participation in an IPE activity may also assist in learning and understanding about profession-specific tasks. Strategies that facilitators can use to increase participation include: (i) motivating the students to become interested through getting them to explore the concept that they 'may not know what they do not know' and, furthermore, (ii) working in the wards alongside the clinicians with whom the students partner, thus gaining credibility with the teams, including medical consultants who then encourage the students to participate in the activity as part of their experience on the ward, and (iii) providing presentations to explain the principles of IPE and the nature of the activity to routine meetings of medical staff.

Facilitators can also address logistical issues such as different curricula and variations in student scheduling through:

- organising a specific time with students to facilitate the desired outcomes, rather than relying on random meeting occasions or assuming that the students will be found on the wards, and
- choosing patients who are under the care of the medical students' consultant so that the patient case is familiar and therefore more likely to be meaningful. In situations where nursing students are placed in a single geographical unit, it is relatively easy to elicit participation of a patient of whom the nursing student has knowledge.

The contribution of a clinical facilitator is important in identifying relevant clinical activities where students can readily engage in interprofessional learning.

8.8.3 Relevant Clinical Activities

Academic staff and clinicians need to give commitment and consideration to effectively structuring learning opportunities for interprofessional practice. Evidence of interprofessional activities is required if the interprofessional activity is to carry meaning for the students (Russell, Nyhof-Young, Abosh, & Robinson, 2006). For example, there are a range of types of activities in which the students could engage: case conferences, team meetings, ward rounds, home visits, and discharge planning (Hilton & Morris, 2001). These kinds of experiences are helpful because they necessarily require groups of medical professionals to come together to discuss patients, their conditions, current treatments, and likely outcomes.

In conjunction with these activities such as team meetings and ward rounds, the proposed activity as outlined is an invaluable resource to guide the sorts of discussions and commence the learning that takes place in more formal interprofessional learning situations. Within the clinical setting, it is important to explore all learning opportunities: medical and nursing students often preferred to keep to themselves and not readily interact with each other in clinical units.

8.9 Summary of Key Considerations for Successful IPE

In summary, leadership across the academic and clinical settings is instrumental in establishing the climate for interprofessional learning. Such a culture supported by leadership exhibits effective communication, collaboration, and teamwork as routine norms of practice. In these circumstances the importance of interprofessional learning is demonstrated to students. Subsequently, relevant clinical situations are created for students to engage in learning across professional groups during the clinical practicum.

8.9.1 Leadership

Leadership across both the university and health sector is essential to plan the curricula and the activities that need to become synonymous with the effective provision of IPE. This leadership gives the mandate for staff to initiate and engage in interprofessional learning. Institutional planning of curriculum and assessment is needed that embeds interprofessional learning and practice throughout the programme of study. Programmes should develop the trajectory of interprofessional competencies around communication and collaboration as detailed, for instance, by the Australian Council for Safety and Quality in Health Care (2005).

Organisational infrastructure that enables students to understand, plan, and participate in interprofessional learning is needed (e.g., clinical placements for medical and nursing students need to be concurrent and within similar geographical locations; interprofessional activities and assessments need to be mandatory for successful completion of the practicum).

8.9.2 Clinician Engagement

At the local level, attention needs to be given to the linking of academic work and clinical activities and, furthermore, the work of the clinicians and the activities that become the everyday routine need to be examined for their potential for interprofessional learning. A number of activities at the local clinical unit level at the interface between staff and students could be implemented to assist with the operation of interprofessional learning, for example:

- Facilitators could work with local teams to encourage them to examine what interprofessional practices they could implement during routine practice.
- In-service sessions, which are routinely undertaken within the professional groups (i.e., medical and nursing students do this separately) could be carefully crafted to engage both nursing and medical students.

Furthermore, consideration could be given to how a facilitator's effects can be optimised, for example, facilitators may receive clarification that their role is:

- To identify interprofessional activities in which students can engage, but not to promote teamwork in the environment (facilitators cannot come from the outside and try and organise team dynamics).
- To identify opportunities, encourage students to interact, and facilitate debriefing and reflective practice.

8.9.3 Relevant Activities

The opportunity to participate in and observe the modelling of interprofessional learning and practice is essential for students to develop good professional practice of their own. While it is recognised that this is not always forthcoming, the benefits of a flexible, self-directed activity can act as a catalyst for the type of learning that is desired in 'real-world' interprofessional practice.

In all, relevant learning activities will emerge from the creation of the learning context through leadership and clinician behaviour that supports the value of health professions collaborating and learning from and with each other.

8.10 Conclusion

It has been proposed here that improving healthcare provisions is premised, in part, on practitioners from distinct professions (e.g., nurses and doctors) coming to communicate and work more effectively together as members of healthcare teams. There is much that inhibits this collaboration, particularly historically derived institutional and occupational practices. There has been little rigorous research around the value of specific clinical placement arrangements and the contribution of the activities in which the students engage during these placements. In response to the kinds of conditions likely to promote effective interprofessional practice and learning, the suggestions provided here are aimed to be instrumental in guiding the investment of commitment, resources, and in-kind support required at all levels of practice from the executive team to the professional group on the floor for such learning to occur within clinical practice settings. The importance of teamwork needs to be introduced early into the curriculum. Moreover, interprofessional learning opportunities that students identify as meaningful and relevant need to be intentionally integrated into the clinical practicum. As identified above, despite the many rigid components of the existing curricula, these types of learning activities can be readily integrated into health professionals' clinical practicums.

Acknowledgements The authors wish to acknowledge the funding support provided through the Australian Learning and Teaching Council's Teaching Fellowship programme.

References

Alexander, H., & Henderson, A. (2010). *Developing a model for interprofessional education during clinical placements for medical and nursing undergraduate students*. Sydney: Australian Learning and Teaching Council.

Anderson, E., Manek, N., & Davidson, A. (2006). Evaluation of a model for maximizing interprofessional education in an acute hospital. *Journal of Interprofessional Care, 20*(2), 182–194.

Australian Commission on Safety and Quality in Healthcare (ACSQHC). (2008). *Clinical handover literature review*. Retrieved July 12, 2010, from www.safetyandquality.gov.au/internet/safety/publishing.nsf/Content/con-clinical-literature

Australian Council for Safety and Quality in Health Care. (2005). *National patient safety educational framework*. Retrieved July 12, 2010, from www.safetyandquality.gov.au/internet/safety/publishing.nsf/Content/60134B7E120C2213CA257483000D8460/$File/npsef_factjul05.pdf

Barker, K. K., Bosco, C., & Oandasan, I. F. (2005). Factors in implementing interprofessional education and collaborative practice initiatives: Findings from key informant interviews. *Journal of Interprofessional Care, 19*(suppl. 1), 166–176.

Barnsteiner, J., Disch, J., Hall, L., Mayer, D., & Moore, S. (2007). Promoting interprofessional education. *Nursing Outlook, 55*(3), 144–150.

Barr, H. (2002). *Interprofessional education: Today, yesterday and tomorrow*. Retrieved June 10, 2010, from http://meds.queensu.ca/quipped/assets/IPE%20Today,%20Yesterday%20&%20Tmmw%20(Barr).pdf

Barr, H., Koppel, I., Reeves, S., Hammick, M., & Freeth, D. (2005). *Effective inter-professional education: Assumption, argument and evidence*. London: Blackwell.

Colyer, H. (2008). Embedding interprofessional learning in pre-registration education in health and social care: Evidence of cultural lag. *Learning in Health and Social Care, 7*(3), 126–133.

Curran, V. R., Sharpe, D., & Forristall, J. (2007). Attitudes of health sciences faculty members towards interprofessional teamwork and education. *Medical Education, 41*(9), 892–896.

Dalton, L., Spencer, J., Dunn, M., Albert, E., Walker, J., & Farrell, G. (2003). Re-thinking approaches to undergraduate health professional education: Interdisciplinary rural placement program. *Collegian, 10*(1), 17–21.

Emerson, T. (2004). Preparing placement supervisors for primary care: An interprofessional perspective from the UK. *Journal of Interprofessional Care, 18*(2), 165–182.

Freeth, D., Hammick, M., Reeves, S., Koppel, I., & Barr, H. (2005). *Effective interprofessional education: Development, delivery and evaluation*. Oxford: Blackwell.

Furber, C., Hickie, J., Lee, K., McLoughlin, A., Boggis, C., Sutton, A., et al. (2004). Interprofessional education in a midwifery curriculum: The learning through the exploration of the professional task project (LEAPT). *Midwifery, 20*(4), 358–366.

Hall, P., & Weaver, L. (2001). Interdisciplinary education and teamwork: A long and winding road. *Medical Education, 35*(9), 867–875.

Hallikainen, J., Väisänen, O., Rosenberg, P. H., Silfvast, T., & Niemi-Murola, L. (2007). Interprofessional education of medical students and paramedics in emergency medicine. *Acta Anaesthesiologica Scandinavica, 51*(3), 372–377.

Hayward, K. S., Kochniuk, L., Powell, L., & Peterson, T. (2005). Changes in students' perceptions of interdisciplinary practice reaching the older adult through mobile service delivery. *Journal of Allied Health, 34*(4), 192–198.

Henderson, A., Twentyman, M., Heel, A., & Lloyd, B. (2006). Students' evaluation of the impact of Clinical Education Units on psycho-social aspects of the clinical learning environment. *Australian Journal of Advanced Nursing, 23*(4), 8–13.

Hilton, R., & Morris, J. (2001). Student placements – Is there evidence supporting team skill development in clinical practice settings?. *Journal of Interprofessional Care, 15*(2), 171–183.

McNair, R., Brown, R., Stone, N., & Sims, J. (2001). Rural interprofessional education: Promoting teamwork in primary health care education and practice. *Australian Journal of Rural Health, 9*(suppl. 1), S19–S26.

Oandasan, I., Baker, G. R., Barker, K., Bosco, C., D'Amour, D., Jones, L., et al. (2006). *Teamwork in healthcare: Promoting effective teamwork in healthcare in Canada*. Ottawa, ON: Canadian Health Services Research Foundation.

Oandasan, I., & Reeves, S. (2005). Key elements for interprofessional education. Part 1: The learner, the educator and the learning context. *Journal of Interprofessional Care, 19*(suppl. 1), 21–38.

Pollard, K. (2009). Student engagement in interprofessional working in practice placement settings. *Journal of Clinical Nursing, 18*(20), 2846–2856.

Reeves, S. (2001). A systematic review of the effects of interprofessional education on staff involved in the care of adults with mental health problems. *Journal of Psychiatric and Mental Health Nursing, 8*(6), 533–542.

Reeves, S., & Freeth, D. (2002). The London training ward: An innovative interprofessional learning initiative. *Journal of Interprofessional Care, 16*(1), 41–52.

Ross, F., & Southgate, L. (2000). Learning together in medical and nursing training: Aspirations and activity. *Medical Education, 34*(9), 739–743.

Russell, K., & Hymans, D. (1999). Interprofessional education for undergraduate students. *Public Health Nursing, 16*(4), 254–262.

Russell, L., Nyhof-Young, J., Abosh, B., & Robinson, S. (2006). An exploratory analysis of an interprofessional learning environment in two hospital clinical teaching units. *Journal of Interprofessional Care, 20*(1), 29–39.

Steinart, Y. (2005). Learning together to teach together: Interprofessional education and faculty development. *Journal of Interprofessional Care, 19*(1), 60–75.

Stone, N. (2007). Coming in from the interprofessional cold in Australia. *Australian Health Review, 31*(3), 332–340.

Thomas, J., Clarke, B., Pollard, K., & Miers, M. (2007). Facilitating interprofessional enquiry-based learning: Dilemmas and strategies. *Journal of Interprofessional Care, 21*(4), 463–465.

Walshe, K., & Offen, N. (2001). A very public failure for quality improvement in health care organisations from the Bristol Royal Infirmary. *Quality in Health Care, 10*(4), 250–256.

Wee, B., Hillier, R., Coles, C., Mountford, B., Sheldon, B., & Turner, P. (2001). Palliative care: A suitable setting for undergraduate interprofessional education. *Palliative Medicine, 15*(6), 487–492.

Young, L., Baker, P., Waller, S., Hodgson, L., & Moor, M. (2007). Knowing your allies: Medical education and interprofessional exposure. *Journal of Interprofessional Care, 21*(2), 155–163.

Chapter 9
Career Development Learning Frameworks for Work-Integrated Learning

Peter McIlveen, Sally Brooks, Anna Lichtenberg, Martin Smith, Peter Torjul, and Joanne Tyler

9.1 Career Development

The meaning of work and career in the contemporary world has undergone significant revision and reformulation as a result of the evolution of work in post-industrial, knowledge economies (Patton & McMahon, 2006). Career has been previously and variously conceptualised in terms of personality types suited to certain work environments, developmental stages, self-efficacy for work behaviours, self-narratives of personal identity, and in terms of personal relationships (McIlveen, 2009). Indeed, a career is more than a job (McMahon & Tatham, 2001) in the contemporary era; *career* can be conceptualised as a multifaceted, complex, personal process that evolves over a person's lifetime, and is influenced by dynamic interactions amongst personal, interpersonal, societal, economic, and environmental factors (Patton & McMahon, 2006). 'Careers are unique to each person and are dynamic: unfolding throughout life. Careers include how persons balance their paid and unpaid work and personal life roles' (Career Industry Council of Australia, 2006, p. 37). This implies a need for individuals to engage in *career self-management* to: (i) participate in lifelong learning supportive of career goals; (ii) locate and effectively use career information; (iii) understand the relationship between work, society, and the economy; (iv) secure/create and maintain work; (v) make career-enhancing decisions; (vi) maintain balanced life and work roles; (vii) understand the changing nature of life and work roles; and (viii) understand, engage in, and manage the career-building process (Ministerial Council on Education Employment Training and Youth Affairs, 2009).

It is within this conceptual remit that we explore the potential of *career development learning* to inform the pedagogy of work-integrated learning. The position advanced here was derived from a major national project that explored the relationship of the two in the context of the Australian higher education system (Smith et al., 2009). Specifically, it is purported that career development learning makes

P. McIlveen (✉)
University of Southern Queensland, Toowoomba, QLD, Australia
e-mail: peter.mcilveen@usq.edu.au

S. Billett, A. Henderson (eds.), *Developing Learning Professionals*, Professional and Practice-based Learning 7, DOI 10.1007/978-90-481-3937-8_9,
© Springer Science+Business Media B.V. 2011

higher education meaningful for students by personalising their learning: enhancing their awareness of the relationships amongst their disciplinary studies, work-related learning, and their personal aspirations. Furthermore, career development learning supports students' effective decision making and transitions into and through the worlds-of-work. Ultimately, we view career development learning through the lens of a philosophy that sees higher education as *growth* (Dewey, 1916); as a developmental process embedded in lifelong learning.

9.2 Career Development Learning in Higher Education

An objective of the project (Smith et al., 2009) was to explore approaches to the delivery of career development learning within the higher education system across some 30 universities in Australia; all of which have a career service of some kind; ordinarily operating as a discrete organisational unit on a university campus; offering the following to services to students:

- advice, support, and delivery of career development learning into the curriculum;
- career assessment and counselling, including selection and change of major;
- career education classes;
- information services relating to occupations, employers, and educational institutions;
- employment placement services for casual, vacation, internship, and graduate employment;
- coordination of employer interviewing;
- operating large-scale employment events (e.g., career fair);
- training on employment application processes (e.g., resumes); and
- academic crisis counselling (e.g., considering dropping out) (Department of Education Employment & Workplace Relations, 2008).

The project discussed here entailed several applied research inquiries. These comprised focus groups and surveys involving university personnel and employers, and interviews of experts to further explore selected cases of practice that demonstrated innovative approaches and excellence. In addition, there was a national symposium on career development learning and work-integrated learning, including career development practitioners, academics, work-integrated learning coordinators, employers, students, professional associations, and government representatives. At this national symposium, participants formulated key themes and principles for effective career service practice. The symposium included discussions from and considerations of literature reviews (McIlveen et al., 2008) and papers delivered by key experts in the field (Barrie, 2008; Kenworthy-U'Ren, 2008; McLennan, 2008; Watts, 2008a, b). The national symposium was followed by a national forum of employers and university students, which further explored and articulated the themes, models, and principles formulated in the national symposium.

Project team members also presented papers and conducted workshops in various national and international forums and conferences to articulate and further refine the themes, models, and principles in response to feedback (e.g., McIlveen et al., 2009a; Smith & Tyler, 2009; Smith, Torjul, Brooks, & Tyler, 2008; Tyler, 2008). Finally, a website was produced to serve as a public repository of resources for students, university staff, and employers. This chapter presents a summary of some of the project's findings, in particular a conceptual framework for career development learning and a graphical model for guiding reflection upon work-integrated learning.

9.3 Alignment of Work-Integrated Learning and Career Development Learning

Although there is no comprehensive and broadly accepted definition of work-integrated learning in the Australian higher education sector (Patrick et al., 2008), a study of the perspectives of university career development practitioners (McIlveen et al., 2009b) found that the description of work-related learning presented by Moreland (2005) was acceptable as a tentative definition of work-integrated learning:

> Work-related learning involves students learning about themselves and the world-of-work in order to empower them to enter and succeed in the world-of-work and their wider lives. Work-related learning involves: learning about oneself; learning and practising skills and personal attributes of value in the world-of-work; experiencing the world-of-work in order to provide insights and learning into the world-of-work associated with one's university studies; and experiencing and learning how to learn and manage oneself in a range of situations, including those found at work. (Moreland, 2005, p. 4)

Moreland's (2005) description of work-related learning furnishes a comparison with career development learning, which can be conceived of as:

> Learning about the content and process of career development or life/career management. The content of career development learning in essence represents learning about self and learning about the world of work. Process learning represents the development of the skills necessary to navigate a successful and satisfying life/career. (McMahon, Patton, & Tatham, 2003, p. 6)

In this way, career development learning focuses on the means by which individuals can successfully manage their lives, learning, and work.

Career development learning occurs in a range of educational and work contexts, and aims to assist students to:

- develop knowledge and understanding of themselves and others as individuals, including the personal resources both actual and potential they bring to situations (i.e., strengths, limitations, abilities, skills, qualities, needs, attitudes, and values);
- develop knowledge and understanding of the general structures of [post-university] life, the range of opportunities and alternative pathways, and the demands, rewards, and satisfaction associated with each;

- learn how to make considered choices and plan options in relation to anticipated careers, occupations, and life roles; and
- effectively manage the implementation of the considered choices and the transitions from [university] to [post-university] situations in adult life and work life (McCowan & McKenzie, 1997, p. 17).

The concordance between career development learning and work-integrated learning is evident in these educational aims. The first of the aforementioned points, for example, can be seen in work-integrated learning practices, such as preparing for and reflecting upon work-related learning experiences. The second and third points may pertain to students' preparation as well as their reflections upon learning whilst in a work environment. The final point exemplifies career development learning and work-integrated learning as means of transition and application of learning for the world-of-work. Essentially, both use work as a crucible for personal development and positive exploitation of higher learning. Towards realising a greater consonance to those ends, we now consider some of the benefits of career development learning.

9.4 Benefits and Scope of Career Development Learning

Career development learning has potential to produce benefits with respect to social equity and human capital (Access Economics, 2006; Hughes, Bosley, Bowes, & Bysshe, 2002; Organisation for Economic Cooperation and Development, 2004; Watts, 2005; Watts, Sweet, Haines, & McMahon, 2006). The benefits of career development learning may be considered from the perspectives of the individual learner; the organisation that employs the individual, and society broadly; and the benefits may accrue within immediate, intermediate, and long-term time frames (Watts, 1999). Immediate benefits may be readily evident and felt by an individual who feels more confident and efficacious with regard to understanding his or her career decisions, plans, and the resources required to implement those plans (e.g., deciding to take a particular degree discipline to become a professional). With regard to the intermediate term, say 6–12 months into a programme of study, as in the previous example, career development learning may provide the benefits of reflecting upon past academic and workplace learning and assimilating new experiences into a burgeoning sense of professional identity; or it may facilitate an individual's accommodation of learning experiences that challenged previously held beliefs or expectations of a degree programme and the profession in sight. In the long term, career development learning may facilitate a sound decision to enter training for a particular profession; alternatively, it may facilitate a decision to adjust career plans and undertake different training pathways for future employability. With regard to the benefits for society-at-large, it is purported that the impact of career development learning upon the individual, multiplied to a societal level, may result in improved student retention and progression in higher education; which can be rendered down to an economic value in terms of public investment in higher education.

The empirical status of career development learning is important for establishing an evidence-based approach to its teaching and facilitating students' learning. There is a considerable and long-standing body of empirical evidence indicating the benefits of career development learning to individuals (Brown & Ryan Krane, 2000; Rochlen, Milburn, & Hill, 2004; Whiston & Oliver, 2005). For example, empirical meta-analytic studies of career development have demonstrated it to be efficacious: with individualised one-on-one career intervention showing the greatest effect size; followed in effect size by career education delivered in a classroom setting; then by the effect of services not delivered by personnel (e.g., ICT delivery) (Whiston, Sexton, & Lasoff, 1998). Longitudinal investigations also indicate a sustained positive impact from individual career guidance (e.g., Bimrose & Barnes, 2006). There is insufficient space to present a review of all of the studies relevant to career development learning; instead, we present a sample of the literature pertaining to two important dimensions of career development learning: engagement with studies and graduate employability. These dimensions were selected because they aligned with the purposes and outcomes of work-integrated learning in higher education.

9.4.1 Engagement with Studies

In relation to work-related learning, engaging in course and career-related employment whilst studying has similarly been found to have positive effects upon academic performance (Derous & Ryan, 2008). Career-related self-efficacy, occupational decidedness, interests, and personality traits have been shown to have a predictive relationship with academic performance and engagement with studies (Brown et al., 2008; Rottinghaus, Lindley, Green, & Borgen, 2002; Sandler, 2000; Scott & Ciani, 2008). Career education coursework, for example, has been found to produce positive outputs: improved career decision-making skills, career decidedness, and vocational identity (Folsom & Reardon, 2003; Fouad, Cotter, & Kantamneni, 2009). Such outcomes assist students to more rationally explore and choose their courses of study and relevant graduate employment options. For example, career development learning has been used to foster first-year undergraduate engineering students' engagement with their studies by assisting them to explore their decision to enter the discipline (Palmer & Bray, 2002); and it has been used to better prepare final-year students for the world-of-work by teaching them skills in self-assessment of employability in relation to current demands in the employment market (Graham, 1999; McIlveen & Gibson, 2000). Folsom and Reardon's (2003) review of 38 empirical studies, conducted over a 25-year period, found evidence of positive effects upon: (i) job satisfaction, (ii) selecting a degree major, (iii) course satisfaction, (iv) retention and graduation rates, and (v) grade-point average. Given that career-related anxiety in undergraduate students is a predictor of academic persistence, career guidance can be implemented as an additional strategy to address student retention and progression (Kahn, Nauta, Gailbreath, Tipps, & Chartrand, 2002).

In summary, the empirical research pertaining to career development learning and engagement with studies provides a platform for our assertion that career development learning can contribute to students making meaningful sense of their higher learning by enabling them to construct relationships amongst their personal aspirations, studies, and experiences of work. It is important also to consider career development learning in terms of its relationship with graduate employability.

9.4.2 Graduate Employability

Cutting across graduate employability, employability skills, and graduate attributes is the notion of lifelong *career self-management* (Bridgstock, 2009; King, 2004), which implies an emphasis upon developing and sustaining individuals' economic viability over their life courses. Indeed, employability skills and graduate attributes may not be entirely sufficient foci for the design of curriculum and programmes in higher learning that effectively engage students' aspirations. Instead, frameworks for the development of personally meaningful career management skills in students (Bridgstock, 2009), such as the *Australian Blueprint for Career Development* (Ministerial Council on Education Employment Training and Youth Affairs, 2009), may present a personally relevant and, therefore, student-centred approach to higher learning and ultimate employability.

Career development learning addresses key issues of *directionality* and *sustainability* of graduate employability (Watts, 2008b); thus, it entails assisting students clarify their career aspirations and how they can manage their progress over time. Career development programmes addressing employability are most notably evident in the delivery of training in employability skills (e.g., McIlveen & Pensiero, 2008) and mentorship programmes (e.g., Theobald, Nancarrow, & McCowan, 1999). There has also been considerable work completed in the application of e-portfolios for the recording of and reflection upon experiences pertaining to employability skills (Colyer & Howell, 2004; Leece, 2005; McCowan, Harper, & Hauville, 2005). These educational initiatives exemplify how career development learning can contribute to improving employability, but it should be noted that career development learning aims for much more than facilitating employability (Bridgstock, 2009); first and foremost, it is fundamental to personal growth and development, and lifelong learning (Patton & McMahon, 2006). Accordingly, from a perspective of the scholarship of teaching and learning it is important that career development learning be linked to conceptual frameworks that can inform curriculum design and evaluation.

9.5 Conceptual Frameworks for Career Development Learning

As part of the project we set out to identify broad conceptual models that could inform the design and delivery of career development learning and work-integrated learning. In this section, we present two frameworks that were constructively modified or generated by participants at the national symposium, and refined by students and employers at their respective national forum.

9.5.1 Domains of Career Development Learning: DOTS Framework

Given the requirement to align or reconcile complexes of factors that comprise the goals for career development learning, it was concluded that the conceptual framework that best satisfied criteria in terms of integration with the world-of-work, self-reflection, and transferability across settings was the DOTS framework (Watts, 2006). We do not assert that the DOTS model is ultimately the best of all purposes; for indeed, there are other approaches that have more extensively artic-ulated career management competencies, such as the eleven competencies in the Australian Blueprint for Career Development (Ministerial Council on Education Employment Training and Youth Affairs, 2009). The DOTS framework was selected for three reasons. First, it has sustained decades of implementation in the higher education sector, particularly in the United Kingdom. Second, DOTS may be rep-resented in a succinct format. Finally, it lends itself to being readily understood and applied by individuals not heavily schooled in the theory of career develop-ment. Four domains comprise the DOTS model: (i) *self-awareness*, (ii) *opportunity awareness*, (iii) *decision making*, and (iv) *transition learning* (Watts, 2006). Both individually and collectively, they provide a framework for organising and ordering career learning. These are now briefly described.

9.5.2 Self-Awareness

The notion of self-awareness is of fundamental to career development learning and reflexivity. According to the DOTS model, self-awareness is comprised of the ability to:

- identify knowledge, abilities, and transferable skills developed by one's degree;
- identify personal skills and how these can be deployed;
- identify one's interests, values, and personality in the context of vocational and life planning;
- identify strengths and weaknesses, and areas requiring further development;
- develop a self-reflective stance to academic work and other activities; and
- synthesise one's key strengths, goals, and motivations into a rounded personal profile (Watts, 2006, pp. 10–11).

Self-awareness underpins students' personal aspirations and selection of courses of study. It contributes to students' relating of disciplinary studies to their pur-poses in undertaking higher education; and it consequently influences students' engagement and progress with studies. For example, self-awareness may contribute to a student's self-appraisal and decision making with regard to which skills he/she needs to enhance whilst participating in a work-integrated learning programme. Career development learning coursework learning activities might include such tasks as completing a self-assessment, using standardised psychometric tools or semi-structured questionnaires, and then the writing of a reflective essay, based upon those self-assessment data, written to a body of disciplinary theory.

9.5.3 Opportunity Awareness

Just as students must be self-aware, they must also be aware of the worlds-of-work if they are to align their interests and energies in an appropriate occupational direction. According to the DOTS model, opportunity awareness requires student to:

- demonstrate knowledge of general trends in graduate employment and opportunities for graduates in one's discipline;
- demonstrate understanding of the requirements of graduate recruiters; and
- demonstrate research-based knowledge of typical degree-related career options and options in which one is interested (Watts, 2006, pp. 10–11).

It would make little sense to a student if a work-integrated learning placement is unrelated to his or her aspirations and learning needs. By being aware of industry trends and requirements, a student is better able to judge the personal relevance and value of a work-integrated learning experience. Thus, a student's awareness of opportunities contributes to how successfully a work-integrated learning experience is rationally considered, secured, and exploited. Coursework learning activities might include students conducting research into the employment market for their particular discipline or a profession to which they aspire by using online search engines, newspapers, or professional newsletters, or conducting interviews with industry recruiters, and then writing a report of their findings with a discussion based upon disciplinary theory.

9.5.4 Decision Making

Self-awareness and understanding opportunities in the worlds-of-work are important, but pragmatically deciding upon directions and actions is quite another thing. Accordingly, the DOTS model stipulates that students can:

- identify the key elements of career decision making in the context of life planning;
- relate self-awareness to knowledge of different opportunities;
- evaluate how personal priorities may impact upon future career options;

- devise a short/medium-term career development action plan;
- identify tactics for addressing the role of chance in career development; and
- review changing plans and ideas on an ongoing basis (Watts, 2006, pp. 10–11).

Decision making builds upon self-awareness and opportunity awareness and pertains directly to actions, such as choosing the most appropriate and valuable work-integrated learning experience. An indiscriminate approach to selecting a learning experience will not effectively serve a student, their site of learning (e.g., workplace), or supervisors. A decision made well will likely prevent negative experiences for all concerned and contribute to students optimally exploiting their work-integrated learning. Coursework learning activities might include the students conducting analyses of case studies in which the career history and decision making of high profile industry experts in a disciplinary field are documented. Their responses to case studies might include speculation on how they might have approached the moments and issues experienced by the individual cases.

9.5.5 Transition Learning

Ultimately, students must progress from the worlds-of-learning to the worlds-of-work, and back again over their lifetimes. The DOTS model requires students not only to understand their direction, but also to make effective transitions from learning to work. They should:

- demonstrate understanding of effective opportunity-search strategies;
- apply understanding of recruitment/selection methods to applications;
- demonstrate ability to use relevant vacancy information, including ways of accessing unadvertised vacancies;
- identify challenges and obstacles to success in obtaining suitable opportunities and strategies for addressing them;
- demonstrate capacity to vary self-presentation to meet requirements of specific opportunities; and
- demonstrate ability to present oneself effectively in selection interviews and other selection processes (Watts, 2006, pp. 10–11).

Graduate employers are increasingly using vacation work or industry experience programmes as pre-recruitment strategies, and work-integrated learning can often align with these experiences (High Fliers Research, 2008). Accordingly, learning how to make successful transitions into placements, particularly if they are situated in a workplace (e.g., formally applying for positions), underpins how students can successfully secure and then retain access to a work-integrated learning placement. Coursework learning activities might build upon aforementioned activities; such as conducting research into the skills required in the employment market for a particular profession and then orally presenting the report of the research findings in class, or via electronic media that can be used to engage other students or prospective employers (e.g., wiki, e-portfolio).

These elements of career development learning may also be considered as cyclical stages, with a person progressively moving through each whilst generating understanding of himself or herself and pragmatic solutions to career-related problems or challenges. A spiral curriculum could be implemented to enable students to advance their understanding and to progressively develop skills associated with each element. Assignments, projects, or other assessable coursework may require students to engage in directed readings, research tasks, journals, or other reflective learning activities in relation to their past, current, and lifelong employability using their particular discipline area of interest as a site of personalised enquiry and self-directed learning. Having just now set out a framework for considering the possible *content* of career development learning and work-integrated learning programmes in terms of the elements the DOTS model, we now turn to a metaphorical model of a *process* of learning: reflection.

9.6 Career Development Learning for Reflective Learning

Career development learning inherently requires a student to (a) engage in processes of self-assessment in terms of individual dimensions (e.g., knowledge, skills, and interests) and (b) perform an appraisal of the context in which the student situates learning in relation to his or her discipline or profession. As a result of it being a personalised pedagogy of self – as a process of self-managed learning and growth – career development learning lends itself to teaching and learning approaches that use reflection in higher learning. The *two-way mirror* shown in Fig. 9.1 depicts the notion of career development learning being used as a mirror for reflection. The two-way mirror concept was initially formulated by participants in the national symposium (Smith et al., 2009). There are three core features of the depiction: the learner, the workplace, and the mirror itself. As the systems theory framework of career development (Patton & McMahon, 2006) suggests, career development learning occurs as a result of a range of influences at the personal level and at the contextual level. At the personal level, individuals' experiences of higher learning are influenced by: self-concept and self-esteem; personality; ethnicity; physical attributes; aptitudes; age; skills; interests; ability; values; sexual orientation; gender; health; disability beliefs; and work knowledge. The personal influences also include peers, home, family, and community, and these are inevitably influenced by the prevailing higher-order external influences: media; employment market; education institutions; workplace legislation; workplace contexts; political decisions; and globalisation. Similarly, a workplace has its own internal influences: organisational structure, expectations, culture, and staff skill sets and behaviour. Workplaces are also influenced by wider community, industry, and government factors. The third feature, career development learning, is the mirror.

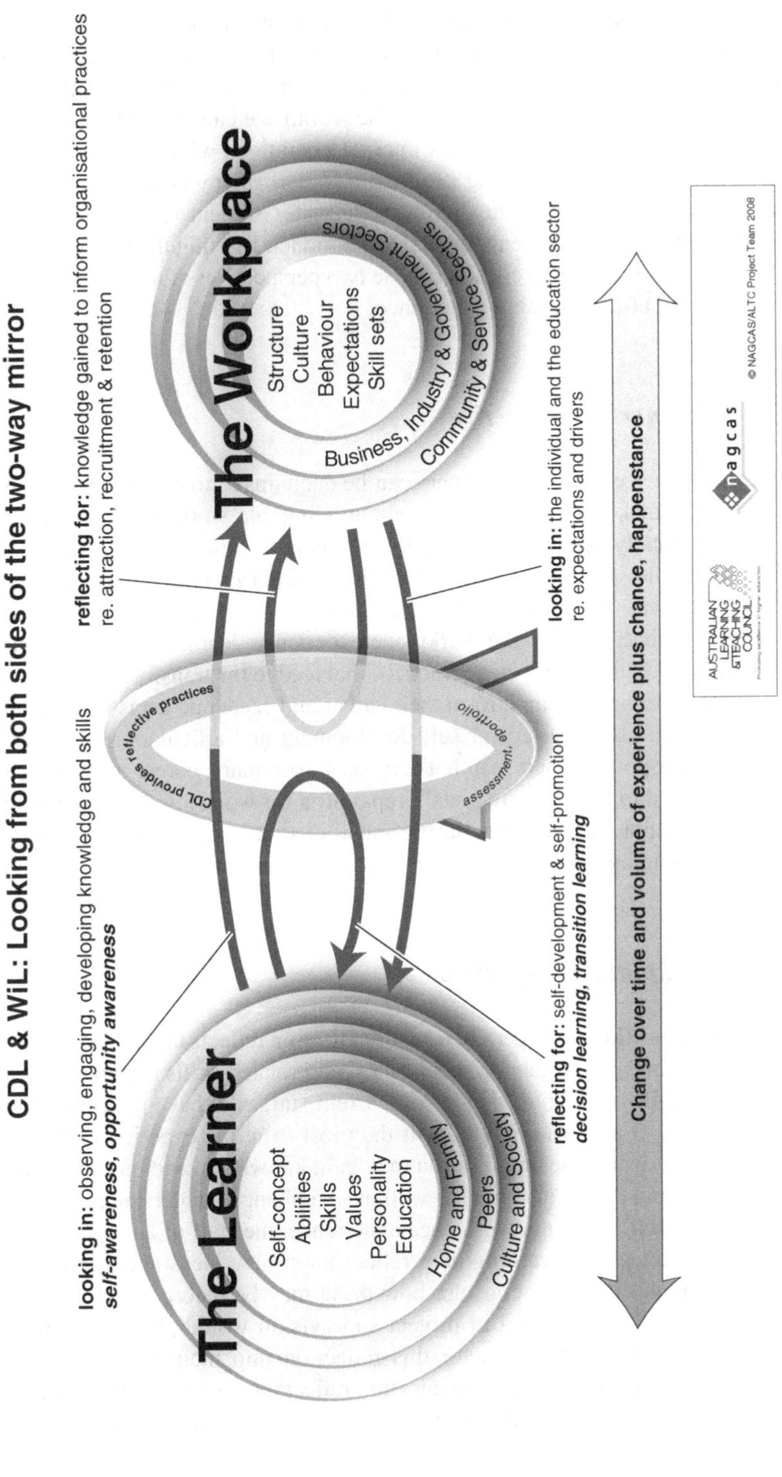

CDL & WiL: Looking from both sides of the two-way mirror

looking in: observing, engaging, developing knowledge and skills
self-awareness, opportunity awareness

reflecting for: knowledge gained to inform organisational practices
re. attraction, recruitment & retention

The Workplace

Government Sectors

Structure
Culture
Behaviour
Expectations
Skill sets

Business, Industry & Govt

Community & Service Sectors

looking in: the individual and the education sector
re. expectations and drivers

CDL provides reflective practices

eportfolio

assessment

The Learner

Self-concept
Abilities
Skills
Values
Personality
Education

Home and Family

Peers

Culture and Society

reflecting for: self-development & self-promotion
decision learning, transition learning

Change over time and volume of experience plus chance, happenstance

© NAGCAS/ALTC Project Team 2008

n a g c a s

AUSTRALIAN
LEARNING
&TEACHING
COUNCIL

Fig. 9.1 Two-way mirror of career development learning and work-integrated learning

There are two perspectives on this mirror: that of the learner and that of the work-place. The learner uses career development learning to reflect upon himself/herself as outlined in the DOTS model previously and in terms of the myriad influences that constitute his/her personal perspective. The workplace can similarly use career development learning to reflect upon its internal operations with regard to how it implements work-integrated learning programmes; perhaps by considering how it establishes a learning environment that best facilitates student learning and staff supervision in terms of the elements in the DOTS model. In using the two-way mir-ror as a metaphor, it is useful to consider those two perspectives at three key stages: before, during, and after a learning experience.

9.6.1 The Learner's Perspective

Before the workplace experience, learners can be encouraged to reflect upon them-selves in order to make informed choices about a suitable workplace experience; that is, to be critically reflexive. During the workplace experience, learners can gain insights into the structure and culture of the workplace and its requisite skills sets and expectations. This can be achieved through observation and engagement in work-related activities. After the workplace experience, learners can be encour-aged and supported in using reflective practices that lead to the transformation of the experience into learning and can inform their career and academic decision making. These practices can also be used for self-development and articulation of experi-ences and skills for potential job search activities. In summary, career development learning can be used to facilitate students' preparation for work-integrated learning, and then to reflect upon their learning during and after so as to exploit the experience as a personally meaningful one.

9.6.2 The Workplace Perspective

Before hosting the workplace experience, an organisation reflects upon their internal contexts, establishing appropriate projects, tasks, and related skills requirements to conduct the activities, as well as identifying current staff who have the right skills to oversee the project and who may benefit the most from the experience. During the workplace experience, the organisation may gain knowledge and understanding of future workers and their capacities, as well as an enhanced understanding of the university sector itself. After the workplace experience, the staff of an organisation involved in work-integrated learning may reflect upon new ideas and approaches brought to the organisation and consider how these may be incorporated in future business processes. Staff involved in project supervision would also reflect upon their own skill development and factor this reflection into their own career and development plans. In addition, the organisation reflects upon knowledge of future workers to inform their attraction, recruitment, and retention strategies. In summary, an organisation can consider the planning, operation, and evaluation of a work-integrated learning programme not only in terms of its impact upon the student, but additionally in terms of how it might improve organisational performance when using work-integrated learning as a pre-recruitment employment strategy (High Fliers Research, 2007).

9.7   Conclusion: Towards Partnerships in Pedagogy

Through an iterative process involving stakeholders in various forums and consultations conducted throughout the national project, a set of principles for practice were developed for the design and delivery of career development learning and work-integrated learning (Smith et al., 2009). These principles capture important practice- and resource-related themes that might shape the effective provision of career learning. The project findings emphasised the value of building and maintaining flexible partnerships amongst stakeholders within universities and industry. Effective relationships and partnerships would serve to increase the range and number of work-integrated learning opportunities and bring stakeholders into a closer understanding of how work-integrated learning is to be taught from their various perspectives. It was concluded that work-related learning experiences can, and should, provide genuine career development learning opportunities for all students, particularly those who may not have ready access to sources of professional networks. Multiple experiences and contexts enrich this learning, and accordingly all forms of work (e.g., voluntary, casual) should be considered as possible sites for work-integrated learning. Career development learning is by its very nature student-centred, and it should be designed to actively engage students in their workplace experience by rendering their work-related learning meaningful in terms of their own career development. Stakeholders also suggested that career development learning supports quality student-centred learning opportunities across all aspects of students' lives, especially given the myriad influences that comprise careers (cf. Patton and McMahon's (2006) systems theory framework). It was also recommended that universities encourage students' career development and workplace learning by supporting their capacity to systematically reflect on, record, and articulate the acquired skills and experience (e.g., portfolios, assessment). Finally, the stakeholders emphasised the importance of developing quality assurance systems for work-integrated learning and career development learning so that all stakeholders were fairly treated in terms of their client-needs.

In this chapter, we have highlighted some of the conceptual dimensions of career development learning that can align with work-integrated learning. In reflecting upon this alignment we concur with Dewey: 'When educators conceive of vocational guidance as something which leads up to a definitive, irretrievable, and complete choice, both education and the chosen vocation are likely to be rigid, hampering further growth' (1916, p. 311). Instead, career development learning should be put to use as means of making higher education personalised, meaningful, relevant, and pragmatically valuable. It should prepare students for the ever-evolving world-of-work, in the sense of enhancing employability, and for a life of learning for personal growth. Furthermore, in this chapter the empirical evidence supporting career development learning's benefits and scope of practices was highlighted to invite consideration of a research agenda for the scholarship of teaching and learning in this field; thus, we conclude with a question: How should career development learning be implemented with curriculum to most effectively exploit its facility as a personally transformative pedagogy, so as to deepen students' engagement with, and improve the learning outcomes derived from, work-integrated learning in higher education?

Acknowledgements This project was conducted by the authors on behalf of the National Association of Graduate Careers Advisory Services (NAGCAS). Support for the original work was provided by the Australian Learning and Teaching Council Ltd., an initiative of the Australian Government Department of Education, Employment and Workplace Relations. The chapter was based upon the final project report: Smith et al. (2009). *Career development learning: Maximising the contribution of work-integrated learning to the student experience. Australian Learning & Teaching Council final project report*. Wollongong: University of Wollongong.

References

Access Economics. (2006). The economic benefits of career development services: Scoping study by Access Economics Pty Ltd for The Career Industry Council of Australia o. Document Number.

Barrie, S. (2008, June 19). *Some ideas about graduate attributes, career development learning and WIL: A preliminary discussion paper*. Paper presented at the National Symposium on Career Development Learning: Maximising the Contribution of Work-integrated Learning (WIL) to the Student Experience, Melbourne.

Bimrose, J., & Barnes, S. (2006). Is career guidance effective? Evidence from a longitudinal study in England. *Australian Journal of Career Development, 15*(2), 19–25.

Bridgstock, R. (2009). The graduate attributes we've overlooked: Enhancing graduate employability through career management skills. *Higher Education Research & Development, 28*(1), 31–44.

Brown, S. D., & Ryan Krane, N. E. (2000). Four (or five) sessions and a cloud of dust: Old assumptions and new observations about career counseling. In S. D. Brown & R. W. Lent (Eds.), *Handbook of counseling psychology* (3rd ed., pp. 740–766). New York: Wiley.

Brown, S. D., Tramayne, S., Hoxha, D., Telander, K., Fan, X., & Lent, R. W. (2008). Social cognitive predictors of college students' academic performance and persistence: A meta-analytic path analysis. *Journal of Vocational Behavior, 72*(3), 298–308.

Career Industry Council of Australia. (2006). *Professional standards for Australian career development practitioners*. Carlton: Author.

Colyer, S., & Howell, J. (2004). An e-portfolio for leisure sciences students: A case study at Edith Cowan University. *Australian Journal of Career Development, 13*(1), 23–32.

Department of Education Employment & Workplace Relations. (2008). Review of career development services in tertiary institutions. Retrieved May 19, 2008, from http://www.deewr.gov.au/

Derous, E., & Ryan, A. M. (2008). When earning is beneficial for learning: The relation of employment and leisure activities to academic outcomes. *Journal of Vocational Behavior, 73*(1), 118–131.

Dewey, J. (1916). *Democracy and education*. New York: The Free Press.

Folsom, B., & Reardon, R. (2003). College career courses: Design and accountability. *Journal of Career Assessment, 11*(4), 421–450.

Fouad, N., Cotter, E. W., & Kantamneni, N. (2009). The effectiveness of a career decision-making course. *Journal of Career Assessment, 17*(3), 338–347.

Graham, C. M. (1999). Career development needs of University engineering students. *Australian Journal of Career Development, 8*(3), 3–7.

High Fliers Research. (2007). *The AAGE graduate recruitment survey 2007*. Melbourne: Australian Association of Graduate Employers Ltd.

High Fliers Research. (2008). *The AAGE employer survey 2008*. Melbourne: Australian Association of Graduate Employers Ltd.

Hughes, D., Bosley, S., Bowes, L., & Bysshe, S. (2002). *The economic benefits of guidance*. Derby: Centre for Guidance Studies, University of Derby.

Kahn, J. H., Nauta, M. M., Gailbreath, R. D., Tipps, J., & Chartrand, J. M. (2002). The utility of career and personality assessment in predicting academic progress. *Journal of Career Assessment, 10*(1), 3–23.

Kenworthy-U'Ren, A. (2008, June 19). *Service-learning and career development learning: A synergistic coupling*. Paper presented at the National Symposium on Career Development Learning: Maximising the Contribution of Work-integrated Learning (WIL) to the Student Experience, Melbourne.

King, Z. (2004). Career self-management: Its nature, causes and consequences. *Journal of Vocational Behavior, 65*(1), 112–133.

Leece, R. (2005). The role of e-portfolios in graduate recruitment. *Australian Journal of Career Development, 14*(2), 72–79.

McCowan, C., Harper, W., & Hauville, K. (2005). Student e-portfolio: The successful implementation of an e-portfolio across a major Australian university. *Australian Journal of Career Development, 14*(2), 40–52.

McCowan, C., & McKenzie, M. (1997). *The guide to career education. For careers personnel working in Australian schools and colleges*. North Sydney, NSW: New Hobsons Press.

McIlveen, P. (2009). Career development, management, and planning from the vocational psychology perspective. In A. Collin & W. Patton (Eds.), *Vocational psychological and organisational perspectives on career: Towards a multidisciplinary dialogue* (pp. 63–89). Rotterdam: Sense Publishers.

McIlveen, P., Brooks, S., Lichtenberg, A., Smith, M., Torjul, P., & Tyler, J. (2008, June 19). *Career development learning & work-integrated learning: A discussion paper*. Paper presented at the National Symposium on Career Development Learning: Maximising the Contribution of Work-integrated Learning (WIL) to the Student Experience, Melbourne.

McIlveen, P., Brooks, S., Lichtenberg, A., Smith, M., Torjul, P., & Tyler, J. (2009a, April 15–17). *Career development learning and work-integrated learning practices in Australian universities*. Paper presented at the Career Development Association of Australia National Career Conference 2009, Melbourne.

McIlveen, P., Brooks, S., Lichtenberg, A., Smith, M., Torjul, P., & Tyler, J. (2009b). Connecting work-integrated learning to the career development DOTS. Submitted for publication.

McIlveen, P., & Gibson, E. (2000). Academic credit and careers education for engineering and surveying students. *Australian Journal of Career Development, 9*(2), 6–7.

McIlveen, P., & Pensiero, D. (2008). Transition of graduates from backpack-to-briefcase: A case study. *Education + Training, 50*(6), 489–499.

McLennan, B. (2008, 19 June). *Work-integrated learning (WIL) in Australian universities: The challenges of mainstreaming WIL*. Paper presented at the National Symposium on Career Development Learning: Maximising the Contribution of Work-integrated Learning (WIL) to the Student Experience, Melbourne.

McMahon, M., Patton, W., & Tatham, P. (2003). *Managing life learning and work in the 21st Century*. Subiaco: Miles Morgan.

McMahon, M., & Tatham, P. (2001). *Career more than just a job*. Canberra, ACT: DETYA.

Ministerial Council on Education Employment Training and Youth Affairs. (2009). The Australian Blueprint for Career Development. Retrieved October 10, 2009, from http://www.blueprint.edu.au/resources/DL_Blueprint_Final.pdf

Moreland, N. (2005). *Work-related learning in higher education*. Heslington, York: The Higher Education Academy.

Organisation for Economic Cooperation and Development. (2004). *Career guidance: A handbook for policy makers*. Paris: Author.

Palmer, S. R., & Bray, S. (2002). An exercise to improve career understanding of commencing engineering and technology students. *Australian Journal of Career Development, 11*(2), 38–44.

Patrick, C. -J., Peach, D., Pocknee, C., Webb, F., Fletcher, M., & Pretto, G. (2008). *The WIL [work-integrated learning] report: A national scoping study*. Retrieved February 12, 2009, from http://www.acen.edu.au

Patton, W., & McMahon, M. (2006). *Career development and systems theory: Connecting theory and practice*. Rotterdam: Sense.

Rochlen, A. B., Milburn, L., & Hill, C. E. (2004). Examining the process and outcome of career counseling for different types of career counseling clients. *Journal of Career Development, 30*, 263–275.

Rottinghaus, P. J., Lindley, L. D., Green, M. A., & Borgen, F. H. (2002). Educational aspirations: The contribution of personality, self-efficacy, and interests. *Journal of Vocational Behavior, 61*(1), 1–19.

Sandler, M. (2000). Career decision-making self-efficacy, perceived stress, and an integrated model of student persistence: A structural model of finances, attitudes, behavior, and career development. *Research in Higher Education, 41*(5), 537–580.

Scott, A. B., & Ciani, K. D. (2008). Effects of an undergraduate career class on men's and women's career decision-making self-efficacy and vocational identity. *Journal of Career Development, 34*(3), 263–285.

Smith, M., Brooks, S., Lichtenberg, A., McIlveen, P., Torjul, P., & Tyler, J. (2009). *Career development learning: Maximising the contribution of work-integrated learning to the student experience. Australian Learning & Teaching Council final project report*. Wollongong, NSW: University of Wollongong.

Smith, M., Torjul, P., Brooks, S., & Tyler, J. (2008, October). *Career development learning: Maximising the contribution of work integrated learning to the student experience*. Paper presented at the ACEN-WACE Asia Pacific Conference, Sydney.

Smith, M., & Tyler, J. (2009, June). *Career development learning: Maximising the contribution of work integrated learning to the student experience*. Paper presented at the WACE World Conference, Vancouver.

Theobald, K., Nancarrow, E., & McCowan, C. (1999). Career mentoring. A career development-enhancing strategy for university students in transition to employment. *Australian Journal of Career Development, 8*(2), 3–7.

Tyler, J. (2008, November). *Internships – graduates making the right choices*. Paper presented at the Australian Association of Graduate Employers Conference Melbourne.

Watts, A. G. (1999). The economic and social benefits of guidance. *Educational and Vocational Guidance Bulletin, 63*, 12–19.

Watts, A. G. (2005). Career guidance policy: An international review. *Career Development Quarterly, 54*(1), 66–76.

Watts, A. G. (2006). *Career development learning and employability*. Heslington, York: The Higher Education Academy.

Watts, A. G. (2008a, 19 June). *Career development learning and work-integrated learning: A conceptual perspective from the UK*. Paper presented at the National Symposium on Career Development Learning: Maximising the Contribution of Work-integrated Learning (WIL) to the Student Experience, Melbourne.

Watts, A. G. (2008b, June 19). *Career development learning and work-integrated learning: Some synthesising reflections*. Paper presented at the National Symposium on Career Development Learning: Maximising the Contribution of Work-integrated Learning (WIL) to the Student Experience, Melbourne.

Watts, A. G., Sweet, R., Haines, C., & McMahon, M. (2006). International symposium on career development and public policy: Synthesis of country papers. *Australian Journal of Career Development, 15*(3), 33–44.

Whiston, S. C., & Oliver, L. W. (2005). Career counseling process and outcome. In M. Savickas &W. B. Walsh (Eds.), *Handbook of vocational psychology: Theory, research, and practice* (3rd ed., pp. 155–194). Mahwah, NJ: Lawrence Erlbaum Associates.

Whiston, S. C., Sexton, T. L., & Lasoff, D. L. (1998). Career-intervention outcome: A replication and extension of Oliver and Spokane (1988). *Journal of Counseling Psychology, 45*, 150–165.

Part II
Institutional Practices and Imperatives

Chapter 10
Scoping Work-Integrated Learning Purposes, Practices and Issues

Deborah Peach and Natalie Gamble

10.1 Promoting Professional Learning Through Work-Integrated Learning: The Australian Context

Currently, there are growing expectations from professional and business communities that university students should be job-ready on graduation. These expectations have led to an increased focus on providing to higher education students experiences that meet these requirements. This chapter draws on the findings of a national scoping study (Patrick et al., 2009) to explore the sources and forms of these demands; and the approaches and models being adopted within Australian higher education to fulfil these demands. It is argued that universities are faced with the challenge of providing opportunities for students to engage in learning experiences connected to the world of work and promoting effective learning for the professional occupations through integrating these experiences into that curriculum. Yet, it would be wrong to view these expectations and these actions as being wholly novel. Indeed, 'There is nothing new in business influencing higher education or in the obsession with skills and employability' (Fearn, 2008, p. 37), nor with responses from universities that involve increased engagement in practice. In Australian higher education, sandwich programmes were first documented as occurring in the late 1940s. These programmes comprised students obtaining a year of professional work experience 'sandwiched' between the second and final year of their university course (Martin, 1997). In the decades since, professional practice programmes have become increasingly popular in university programmes with a specific occupational focus, including nursing, teaching and engineering. These approaches to educational practice have also been widely adopted in programmes of study not traditionally associated with the trades and college-based professions. Those adopting these kinds of approaches include the business, science and creative arts areas of study. In the late 1980s, government and industry began placing increasing demands on Australian higher education providers to develop more occupationally

D. Peach (✉)
Queensland University of Technology, Brisbane, QLD, Australia
e-mail: d.peach@qut.edu.au

S. Billett, A. Henderson (eds.), *Developing Learning Professionals*, Professional
and Practice-based Learning 7, DOI 10.1007/978-90-481-3937-8_10,
© Springer Science+Business Media B.V. 2011

relevant and equitable curriculum, with an emphasis on aligning what is learnt in university programmes with the reality of workplaces in which graduates would practice (Department of Education, Employment and Workplace Relations (DEET), 1990). This emphasis has continued and a consideration of providing experiences in practice settings has intensified.

However, what has changed in the past two decades is the massification of higher education and the introduction of a user-pays system. University students (now in larger numbers) are both pressed and responding eagerly to complete their degree programmes in as short a time as possible to start earning and avoid accruing more educational debt. Universities are also under pressure in an increasingly competitive environment to demonstrate the relevance of their courses and accountability and effectiveness in their use of tax payer funds, whilst also being responsive to the needs of fee-paying students. These pressures have led to an emphasis on graduating work-ready students with both broadly applicable employment skills and abilities and occupationally specific knowledge and understanding. A particular consequence of all this has been an increased interest in Work-Integrated Learning (WIL) – providing and integrating experiences in both practice and university settings – and the role it plays in preparing students for the workforce, developing graduate attributes, improving graduate employability and meeting economic imperatives and, more recently, building greater diversity and social participation (Bradley, Noonan, Nugent, & Scales, 2008; Department of Education, Employment and Workplace Relations (DEEWR, 2009). Indeed, the demands referred to above have led to a questioning of the kinds of experiences that university programmes provide, and the role of universities in preparing students and graduates for specific occupations. It is on these issues of promoting effective learning for the professions that this chapter focuses. In doing so, it refers to the growing demand for capacities that promote graduates' employability. That is, it is claimed that these expectations are growing and demanding new roles of study within higher education. However, as universities engage in these new roles, they may well require guidance in how best they can fulfil these emerging obligations to their students and community. To provide some models and approaches, the outcomes of a scoping study which gathered information about the range of practices being adopted are used as a basis for offering options and alternatives for practice within universities. In considering which approaches and practices are most relevant to particular areas, it is proposed that the specific educational worth of providing students with practicum experiences needs to be considered. From this, some approaches and models are advanced as a means of suggesting how institutional responses might progress in addressing these emerging requirements.

10.2 Emerging Student Demands for Higher Education Programmes

As noted, there is nothing particularly novel about professional and business communities making demands upon higher education (Consortium for Integrated Resource Management (CIRM), 2008; Maher & Graves, 2008). However, as a result of changes in policies, particularly a user-pays system of higher education, a new set of demands is being directed towards the sector. Yet, there are tensions between the expectations of the community about the kinds of programmes that will be offered and how they will be offered, on the one hand, and what universities are able and prepared to offer, on the other. In particular, it seems that university students are increasingly demanding an experience directly relevant to their future employment aspirations and that can also provide personal and positional advantage, especially in a period of economic downturn and lack of employment security (Precision Consultancy, 2007; The Panel on Fair Access to the Professions, 2009; Universities Australia, 2008). That is, students want experiences that are practice-oriented to develop occupationally specific and employable capacities. According to an analysis of open-ended comments from over 94,000 students from 14 Australian universities, students want a 'total experience of university not just what happens in the traditional classroom' (Scott, 2005, p. vii). The analysis of over 160,000 comments gathered between 2001 and 2004 via the national Course Experience Questionnaire (CEQ) also indicates that students claim they value highly relevant, practical experiences and they are motivated by learning experiences that are relevant, desirable, distinctive and achievable. This, of course, is an understandable set of expectations from students to engage increasingly in occupationally specific educational programmes. These expectations also appear to be quite enduring.

A 2008 review of student engagement over time with learning and teaching in Australian higher education (Scott, 2008) claims, again, that these kinds of expectations of university study outcomes have always existed and are likely to be common to most student groups, and across both international and domestic students. Scott's study found students expect that university studies will have personal and vocational relevance, that there will be coherence in what is studied and assessed, and that the totality of their experiences will provide them with the capacities to be employed in their selected occupation upon graduation. Hence, students have long held expectations about the relevance of their studies to their future aspirations; the extent to which universities will be clear about what is available; and the provision of sound, timely and responsive advice when choosing programmes of study. However, with the advent of direct or indirect fee payments, students have growing expectations about the delivery of what is promised; and that social experiences and support they access will be positive; easy access to responsive and skilled teachers will be available; that assessment requirements are clear; and they will receive timely and constructive feedback on their assessment tasks (Thurgate & MacGregor, 2009). Increasingly, students also expect targeted and sustained assistance with transition into the university culture, especially for those who are the first in their family to attend university, and then from there into the world of work, and in particular, their selected occupation upon graduation. All of these expectations make for very demanding educational goals and processes, of which the provision of WIL experiences is a part.

However, whilst increasingly clear and strong in their expectations, students may not be well positioned to judge what will prove to be the most relevant educational experiences. This is because most likely they do not yet fully understand the requirements of their selected profession, and its application in settings where they will actually seek employment. Nevertheless, universities are inheriting an obligation to focus more on addressing students' needs, aspirations, motivations and distinct profiles; provide programmes of interest to individual students; make programmes relevant to individual needs and purposes; and help students develop the capacities required for competent practice (Carapinha, 2007). For instance, a 2008 Carnegie Foundation project (Sullivan & Rosin, 2008) found the focus of higher education should be on the development of graduates capable of negotiating effectively the combined set of social, ethical, intellectual and technical challenges within their chosen profession or discipline. This again is highly ambitious given the diverse circumstances in which the practice of teaching, nursing or engineering, for instance, is enacted. Indeed, the increased focus on social and ethical issues is seen as not only enhancing professional and disciplinary performance, but as having much broader societal benefits These claims may or may not be aligned with contemporary student demands of higher education, but they highlight the need to consider the changing expectations of higher education in an increasingly diverse and global workplace (Sullivan & Rosin, 2008).

Moreover, other changes in the operating environment of universities have generated a range of additional student expectations that are now required to be fulfilled. For example, the increasing diversity of the student body makes the mix of expectations more complex – including the likelihood that some students will have expectations that are too high, too low or which are uninformed. With more full-time students concurrently working, expectations about flexible, responsive and cost-effective study modes are increasing. Similarly, with rising costs of higher education, students are increasingly focusing on making sure they get 'value for money'. The effective use of technology as part of a broader learning experience is also anticipated along with direct, up-front assistance on how to use the technology (Scott, 2008). In all, these forms of highly self-directed support bring additional requirements for students to be ready to engage effectively with such technology.

Given all of these requirements, it is helpful to know that when the demands of students for work experiences are met, these are reported as being highly useful for them. Research in Australia (Precision Consultancy, 2007; Universities Australia, 2008), the United States (Cates & Cedercreutz, 2008; Gardner, 2008; Sullivan & Rosin, 2008) and the United Kingdom (Maher & Graves, 2008) concludes that students who had undertaken a work experience or a skill development component as part of their higher education programme were more likely to view their university experience positively and go on to secure employment within their chosen field than those students not having had these experiences. Yet, Australian universities are being challenged by the gap between what students and employers want and what universities are able and/or willing to deliver, and by the difficulties of measuring the quality of learning experiences that do not necessarily fit with existing models of learning and teaching. For instance, a discussion paper by a higher education peak body (Universities Australia, 2008) points to the need to balance university mission (i.e. to produce graduates who are well educated, fully employable and who are critical, creative, sharp thinkers with emotional intelligence) with market demands (i.e. an instrumental, vocational focus). Consequently, there are ongoing tensions amongst the beliefs and values of industry, the community and students about the kinds of educational purposes that universities should serve.

The aim of pointing out these tensions is to optimise the quality of every student's experience without compromising the quality and credibility of university study. Universities Australia (2008) proposes further enhancement of work-ready skills especially in a structured way that complements and enhances more general learning outcomes. These experiences across different kinds of programmes will be served by better understanding educational purpose. Also, given the diversity of ways in which such an agenda might be addressed, it is worthwhile scoping a range of practices used across the sector in responding to these demands. Consequently, all of this suggests that in considering WIL as a key element of the higher education provision, it is important that programmes are able to address a range of educational purposes. These include assisting the development of occupationally specific capacities, whilst at the same time generating the kinds of learning outcomes which are seen to be not only more broadly applicable but also able to assist graduates engage thoughtfully and critically with issues and problems both within their selected occupations and outside of them. In the next section consideration is given to the ways in which work experiences are being positioned in university programmes and how they might achieve some of these ambitious goals.

10.3 Scoping Work Experience Practices

One aim of seeking to understand how universities provide work experience is to ascertain something of the range of conceptions and approaches and to understand their particular educational utility and potential to be applied elsewhere. Earlier, Australian research focused predominantly on specific models, pedagogical or theoretical issues, or stakeholder perspectives, such as those of students and employers (see Atchison, Pollock, Reeders, & Rizzetti, 2002; Cooper, Orrell, & Jones, 1999). However, the account provided here draws largely upon a national study to capture the scope of these practices across Australian higher education (Patrick et al., 2009). The aim of this study was to inform the development of effective and innovative curriculum to improve student learning through the provision of practice-based experiences. The study process comprised mapping existing practices, issues and challenges within Australian higher education to inform policy-makers, researchers, academic and professional staff, and other stakeholders involved in decision making about WIL.

The study utilised a broad-based networking strategy to engage participants and gather data about WIL practices across nearly all Australian higher education institutions. Participants included university students and staff, employers and representatives of state and federal government. However, access to these participants was uneven due to availability and some perspectives were more readily captured than others. For example, university academic and professional staff widely participated. Gaining access to students was dependent upon the cooperation of participating universities, and proceeded unevenly. Similarly, employer/community perspectives were similarly constrained and government input was mainly via relevant reports. Nevertheless, a rich description of the practices, issues and challenges faced by stakeholders across a range of disciplines was secured through this study. In the following sections, conceptions of providing learning experiences connected to work, the worth of these experiences, and related challenges are progressed. A discussion about the character and qualities of these experiences progresses largely through a review of literature. Considerations of educational worth also arise through literature, and accounts of practice through focus group and interview activities. The challenges that emerge from an analysis of project data provide universities with a starting point to confront the prospect of providing a range of opportunities that afford effective learning for the professions.

10.4 Conceptions of Providing Learning Experiences Connected to Work

Different concepts are used in Australian higher education to describe the learning approaches and teaching models providing students with opportunities to engage in learning experiences as part of work. These experiences are sometimes presented as 'real world learning' or 'professional learning' with others preferring the term 'community engagement'. At another level, terms such as fieldwork, practicum, clinical placement, industry-based learning, sandwich years, cooperative education, work placements and internships are used to describe methods universities use to equip students with knowledge of workplace practices. Often these terms arise from the particular field of practice. Hence, reference to clinical experiences or practices tends to be derived from healthcare occupations whereas a term such as fieldwork likely has different origins. Discussion has continued over time about terminology and naming conventions and these issues sometimes arise for educational institutions when the same kinds of experiences are referred to by different names, and when different experiences are referred to by the same name (Calway, 2006; Martin, 1998; Smigiel & Harris, 2007). Nevertheless, despite the differences in their origins and naming, these approaches are often collectively referred to as WIL with an understanding that they share common features such as:

1. being based on identified industry needs and expectations of graduates and employees (for example, professional accreditation), which are integrated into the curriculum;
2. inclusion of the work component as part of the overall curriculum design;
3. involvement of industry partners who, in addition to providing advice on curriculum design, also provide workplaces for students to gain experience; and

4. a formal system which supports students and provides a framework for organising and assessing student work and experience (Precision Consultancy, 2007, p. 29).

A trigger for many universities to change the structure and naming conventions of existing WIL programmes was provided in 2005 by the federal government. Policy changes to the Commonwealth Grant Scheme (CGS)[1] forced universities to focus attention on the level of oversight, direction and management of student learning provided through learning experiences connected to work (especially work placement programmes). The Higher Education Support Act (HESA) Administrative Guidelines (DEEWR, 2008) specify that student learning and performance is directed by the provider (that is, the university) if all of the following are performed by the provider or persons engaged by the provider:

- ongoing and regular input and contact with students;
- oversight and direction of work occurring during its performance, not just regarding the progress of a student's work;
- definition and management of the implementation of educational content and objectives of the unit;
- definition and management of assessment of student learning and performance during the placement; and
- definition and management of the standard of learning.

The HESA Administrative Guidelines (DEEWR, 2008) also specify that student learning and performance is supported if the provider: initiates interaction between the supervisor and the student, which may include site visits; organises student placements; monitors student work and progress (ongoing); and assesses student learning and performance during the placement. Whilst these are guidelines only and universities may well interpret them differently, the outcome of these policy changes has been an increased awareness of and interest in the way work-related learning experiences are described and implemented, and has done much to precipitate the need for a shared terminology.

For its purposes, the WIL Report (Patrick et al., 2009, p. 9) defines WIL as 'an umbrella term for a range of approaches and strategies that integrate theory with the practice of work within a purposefully designed curriculum'. When the project commenced issues around terminology were still very relevant. However, early on the project team were advised to avoid working towards a definition of work-integrated learning for the purposes of discriminating between approaches that would be included in, or excluded from, the study. Instead, the study identified a wide range of terms actively being used by universities that would fall under

---

[1] The Commonwealth Grant Scheme (CGS) provides funding and support for an agreed number of undergraduate higher education places at each Australian tertiary institution in a given year, subject to a funding agreement with the Commonwealth.

Table 10.1 WIL terminology: Frequency of use (derived from Patrick et al., 2009)

Rank	Term/s (frequency)
1	Practicum (35)
2	Professional practice (32)
3	Internship, workplace learning, work-integrated learning (31)
4	Industry-based learning (25)
5	Project-based learning (24)
6	Cooperative education, fieldwork education (20)
7	Service learning (12)
8	Real world learning (9)
9	University engaged learning (7)
10	Placements (6)
11	Experiential learning (5)
12	Clinical placements, professional placement (4)
13	Work experience (3)
14	Clinical practice, clinical education, doctoral supervision with industry partners, work-based learning (2)
15	Academic service learning, adult learning, andragogy, clinical attachments, clinical experience, competency assessment, corporate business management, employment experience, engaged learning, experiential placements, faculty internships, field placements, industrial experience, industry experience, industry links, industry placement, learning in the workplace, operational performance, practical projects, practical training, practice-based education, problem-based learning, professional experience, professional learning, sandwich, site visits, structured workplace learning, student employability, volunteering (1)

the project's broad definition. These terms numbered 47 in all (see Table 10.1). Table 10.1 ranks the frequency of terms identified in survey, interview and focus group data, and the figures in brackets indicate the number of times the term was used.

As can be seen in Table 10.1, the most commonly reported term used to describe work-related learning experiences was 'practicum', a term closely associated with teacher education, nursing, social work and allied health, but even these disciplines are likely to refer to it in a variety of ways such as clinical placement, teaching rounds, or professional practice. Other frequently used terms included professional practice, internships, workplace learning, industry-based learning, project-based learning and cooperative education. It is important to understand that many of these terms are well embedded in the practice of disciplinary areas within universities, and also their external partners. Regardless of the term/s used, it is important to highlight that the priority here, and educationally, is to identify and secure the kinds of experiences that will assist students' learning, not what these experiences are called.

One interpretation of Table 10.1 is that WIL is healthy and thriving in the Australian university sector, and is manifesting itself in a multitude of named learning and teaching practices. It also illustrates the problems created by varied naming conventions These problems include difficulties in measuring outcomes when terminology is not commonly understood and consequent implications for policy and resourcing (Smigiel & Harris, 2007). Additionally, terminology impacts on quality assurance and on an institution's ability to accurately report on WIL activities. For instance, one institution has embedded a variety of terms associated with both on- and off-campus WIL practices in its revised policy for the purposes of improved tracking and reporting in response to the HESA Administrative Guidelines (DEEWR, 2008). The point here is that the particular approach taken by individual institutions in addressing growing governmental and community demands and student expectations will be premised on a range of historical and institutional preferences. For instance, some may seek to downplay the emphasis on highly applied studies, to maintain a profile that emphasises more general learning outcomes. Or, as is more likely, the approach and terminology will be carefully tailored to the kinds of goals which the institutions seek to realise.

The decision by the Australian federal governments to fund only those programmes that direct and support students' learning experience in the workplace acknowledges that work experience itself is not necessarily intrinsically beneficial. Therefore, some particular kinds of work-related experiences are likely to be seen as being more legitimate than others. In particular, those experiences which comprise supervised placement are often seen as being the most legitimate and worthwhile. This view is consistent with the findings of Knight and Yorke (2004), who report that work experience without adequate support from higher education providers does little for student learning. Moreover, these authors also claim that intentional, organised and recognised educational experiences that provide meaningful engagement with the workplace have the potential to greatly enhance a student's work readiness and their employment opportunities. More importantly, whatever the terminology used it is imperative that students have a clear understanding of the learning outcomes and expectations of their WIL experience and that institutions find ways to present a coherent interpretation to stakeholders that supports effective learning for the professions (Patrick et al., 2009). In these ways, fulfilling the expectations of both students and community might require levels of engagement in a range of future occupations which do not currently exist. Opening up such arrangements is likely to be a long-term process and one requiring significant funding for it to be more broadly applied. In the context of these conceptions of WIL, its educational worth is discussed in the next section.

10.5 The Educational Worth of WIL

Much of what has been published on WIL emphasises the benefits for each of the key stakeholders: students, industry hosts and universities. It is likely that all of these benefits are premised on WIL's educational worth, albeit in slightly different ways. One view is that worth is through the development of so-called generic employability skills and capabilities that assist graduates to be effective in paid employment, regardless of specific occupational and workplace requirements. From this perspective, a key objective of WIL is to consolidate and complement academic learning, knowledge and skills, while integrating some aspects of personal career awareness and development (Smith et al., 2009). This latter set of learnings is sometimes referred to as career development learning (McMahon, Patton, & Tatham, 2003), and involves students learning about themselves, and the way they interact with the world of work. There are other benefits associated with the development of occupationally specific capacities. As noted above, many view such learning as being not worthy of higher education unless criticality and analytical capacities of a generally applicable kind are also developed. So, given these distinct bases for making judgements about worthiness, we need ways to evaluate the educational worth of WIL.

Conceptions of how WIL might be best valued also draw on a number of learning theories and pedagogies, including experiential-based learning, immersive learning and transformative learning (Andresen, Boud, & Cohen, 1995; Kolb, 1984; Mezirow, 1997). For example, features of experiential-based learning, such as involvement of the whole person; recognition and use of life experiences; and continued reflection on learning, underpin the perceived worth of work-related learning experiences. In all, WIL should be viewed as an integrated learning process, shaped by the characteristics of the individual and their interactions with the work environment (Marsick, 2009). Further, it should give students the opportunity to 'learn by doing', as they are immersed in a workplace or simulated work environment. That is, WIL has the potential to provide students with the opportunity to bring theory and practice together and to make sense of their experiences, through reflective, transformative practices. In this way, WIL can be seen as an active, student-centred approach to learning that is embedded in curriculum in such a way that it complements students' levels of theory and knowledge attainment and enhances skills that students acquire through application and reflection. In accordance with curriculum design principles, it follows that learning experiences connected to the world of work should become increasingly demanding as students progress and their understanding of their discipline deepens along with a sense of an emerging professional identity. For instance, O'Shea (2009) suggests that experiences over the course of a degree should start with less demanding classroom-based scenarios, and culminate in high level activities and projects that occur in the workplace.

Workplaces, as learning environments, may well provide students with opportunities to integrate theory and practice, and to reflect on the world of work while gaining a cultural awareness of the discipline or field. Because students are required to engage in activities and interactions they are required to apply what they have learnt earlier to what they encounter in the work or practice setting. Billett (2001, p. 2) observes that 'social situations, such as workplaces, are not just one-off sources of learning and knowing. Instead, they constitute environments in which knowing and learning are co-constructed through ongoing and reciprocal processes'. He suggests that there 'is long-standing evidence of the efficacy of learning in the workplace' (Billett, 2001, p. 19). That is, workplace learning has the potential to provide students with the opportunity to demonstrate their understanding in authentic and meaningful contexts.

Realising this potential requires quality preparation and the articulation of clear expectations that are understood by all stakeholders. Harvey, Moon, and Geall (1997) argue that the quality of the learning experience is tied to its relevance, structure, organisation and intentionality. University staff who participated in the national scoping study cited adequate preparation, appropriate supervision and mentoring arrangements as crucial components of effective WIL strategies. As one survey respondent stated, 'There is a need for pre-placement, during placement and post placement coherence so that students are adequately prepared for placement, with supervisors considering these various phases and the skills and the preparation needed' (Patrick et al., 2009). Participants also highlighted the importance of clarifying expectations, and linked this with effective supervision: 'Ensuring the match between student expectations and workplace expectations. Making sure both (are) prepared for the WIL so (the) relationship (is) positive' (Patrick et al., 2009).

Building on the kinds of comments advanced above, an emerging area of interest is the identification of an effective WIL pedagogy that provides a transformative learning experience for students that crosses university and workplace boundaries (Savage, 2005; Davis, Franz, & Plakalovic, 2009). This pedagogy likely requires that learners are assisted to become aware and critical of their own and others' assumptions and engage in 'recognising frames of reference and using their imaginations to redefine problems from a different perspective' (Mezirow, 1997, p. 10). That is, learning experiences are required that involve a concerted, integrated approach to developing students' academic skills, encouraging critical reflective learning and the ability to reflect and articulate what has been learnt.

Billett (2009) argues that professional practitioners are required to be agentic (i.e. to be intentional, directed and critical in their practice). This capacity is also central to their learning to become a practitioner. This requirement points to the need for universities to identify ways of developing criticality, personal agency and self-direction in students through intentionally designed and facilitated curriculum and pedagogy. Andresen et al. (1995) agree that much of the impetus for experience-based learning has been a reaction against an approach to learning which is overly didactic, teacher controlled and involving a discipline-constrained transmission of knowledge. WIL supports a more participative, learner-centred approach, which places an emphasis on direct engagement, rich learning events and the construction of meaning by agentic learners. These qualities are quite distinct from a didactic pedagogy.

Informants from many of the universities participating in the scoping study reported actively seeking ways to integrate work-based learning experiences across the whole of curriculum and incorporate sequential teaching and assessment approaches from first to final year that incorporate these experiences. The informants emphasised that WIL is more than 'just placements' and this is reflected in the broad range of approaches adopted by these informants' disciplines, including work placements, project work and simulations. However, there appear to be tensions amongst what one respondent described as 'the employer objectives and academic objectives' and 'generic skills objectives within the curriculum and more discipline-specific skills'. Some academic staff indicated the potential for mismatched ideologies between 'academe and workplace, that is, learning versus working; holistic care versus task-based care; altruism versus economics' (Patrick et al., 2009). Nevertheless, other senior management and academic staff emphasised the importance of balancing differing objectives which can be complementary. Another respondent observed that there was a 'synergy between the two – knowledge and life skills', while another saw WIL as playing a role in 'adequately preparing students for the experience of a balance of academia and work skills' (Patrick et al., 2009). In summary, the educational worth of WIL is premised upon the particular orientation the evaluator adopts, yet there are conceptual premises that can legitimate these orientations from a number of theoretical perspectives. The particular orientations also shape how WIL is enacted. Some of the instances and models are described below.

10.6 Instances/Models of Practice

Although still associated predominantly with situated work placements, WIL is now seen as encompassing far more than learning experiences that occur in the workplace. In Australia, currently, many universities are making a concerted effort to embed WIL across disciplines and in doing so expose students to a spectrum of learning opportunities that have relevance in the worlds beyond universities. Alternatives to work placements include project and problem-based learning, teaching through rich case studies, and simulations. That is, learning experiences previously associated with work placements are now being reproduced in classroom environments through these approaches as well as those identified in case studies as part of the scoping study (Australian Learning and Teaching Council, 2010). These cases represent some snapshots of the broad range of possible practice and highlight different perspectives and practical implications. The case studies include instances of internships, practicum, field projects and virtual placements. For example, a virtual placement programme offered to law students at one university provides students with the opportunity to contribute to 'real' cases in a virtual environment. An alternative to the virtual placement is the fully immersive workplace experience, such as that offered to science, environment, engineering and technology students. This approach provides students with structured support systems, which facilitate professional growth and skill acquisition through project work. This diversity and flexibility of models and approaches should be recognised, articulated and used to illustrate how some disciplines innovate and adapt to meet the particular needs of students, industry partners and disciplines. The case studies illustrate not only the distinct traditions across disciplines but also that the universities canvassed in the study are quite flexible, adaptive, scholarly and innovative in their approach to curriculum design.

However, further systematic work still needs to be undertaken to identify the full range and breadth of programmes available, their educational purpose and the learning outcomes achieved by students who participate. Strategies for linking the significant body of knowledge about learning experience connected to work in disciplines such as education, nursing, engineering and medicine, to new and evolving programmes would be worthwhile. This will require extensive effort because, as highlighted earlier, many disciplines do not readily identify themselves with terminology such as WIL, cooperative education or placements. Regardless of the terminology used, the notion of authenticity is of critical importance in order to maximise learning outcomes from the learning experiences, as is the level of planning and support provided by universities; the effort that goes into the design and development of the activities is usually indicative of the value associated with WIL. To conclude, some of the challenges that these efforts present universities trying to increase student participation and improve learning outcomes are discussed briefly.

10.7 Issues That Impact on Quality and Access

If universities are to respond to student needs and demands for more relevant curriculum that provides effective learning for the professions they must address several key challenges. The scoping study identified challenges or issues related to equity and access, expectations and competing demands, improved communication and coordination, ensuring worthwhile placement experiences, and adequate resourcing. The study recognises that not all students have easy or equal access to WIL, even where it is mandated for professional accreditation. For example, some international students struggle to find placements, and students with family and/or financial responsibilities may not be in a position to pursue opportunities, particularly where they are unpaid. A UK study recommends that WIL programmes adhere to a minimum set of standards, encouraging employers to implement quality, equitable internship programmes and ensuring that participation is affordable for all students; and provides information and advice on how such standards may be achieved (The Panel on Fair Access to the Professions, 2009). The Australian scoping study also highlights the practice in some programmes of restricting access to these kinds of experiences to only high-achieving students. Whilst this practice may benefit the employer and help showcase the university, it is also the case that less academically able students, or those who are not necessarily academic high achievers, often benefit most from the developmental opportunities afforded by learning experiences connected to the world of work (Edwards, 2007; Precision Consultancy, 2007). As one participant in the scoping study observed: 'Judging whether a student is prepared involves more than just academic results and includes communication skills, interpersonal skills, and a good attitude because a lot of the technical skills are learned on the job. Universities need to take this into account' (Patrick et al., 2009). If WIL is to become an even stronger feature of university curriculum, then consideration must be given to issues of widening participation and associated costs to individuals, industry hosts and institutions. Fulfilling such expectations raises another tension regarding the capacity to locate appropriate and sufficient placements.

There are often 'expectation gaps' when stakeholders have different motivations and different reasons for engaging with WIL. A distinguishing feature of effective programmes is that they involve partnerships among diverse groups: university students and staff, industry partners, professional bodies, and broker agencies such as careers services and external placement groups (Orrell, 2004). However, having partnerships able to meet and sustain expectations held by students, employers and universities may not be easy. Calway (2006) claims that student expectations include: securing enhanced employability, developing marketable job skills, exposure to current practices and clarification of career goals. Almost contrarily, this study also found that many employers engage with WIL anticipating high levels of student competence, the ability to successfully complete project work, securing workers at a lower cost, the opportunity to identify and train a possible future employee, access to (latest) university practice, and the benefit of having access to up-to-date knowledge. It is easy to see here how expectations might be challenged on both sides. Universities, it seems, are held to pursue WIL with the expectation that the experience will help produce workforce-ready students, enhance the reputation of the university, increase graduate employability, strengthen partnerships with industry and yield high measures of student satisfaction. Again, anticipating possible misapprehensions between students and employers, it is possible that the purposes universities intend may not be forthcoming. Patrick et al. (2009) suggest a 'stakeholder-integrated approach' based on formalised partnerships with a common understanding is required to minimise conflict and to maximise learning outcomes. The report also highlights that students and employers need to be aware of limitations on both sides during placements and to be realistic regarding what can be achieved. The evidence from this study suggests that universities must be aware of students' levels of workplace knowledge, for example, if they have worked before and their knowledge of work ethics, prior to engaging in workplace-related learning experiences. Some students may require an induction and/or 'refresher' on the basics before getting fully involved in their placement tasks. Putting unprepared and inadequately supervised students in the workplace was seen as a potentially risky and an educationally and institutionally counter-productive process, as can be imagined on the basis of the misaligned expectations outlined above.

Across Australian universities it was found that the nature and quality of the relationships between students, host organisations and universities is indicative of the quality of the student-learning outcomes. Responses highlight the importance of strong partnerships between stakeholders to facilitate effective learning outcomes and a range of issues that shape the quality of learning purposes, practices and outcomes. Open dialogue is most likely to lead to sustainable and mutually beneficial experiences for all involved. The study's findings also highlight the importance of having access to relevant information about various approaches and identify that good coordination and communication is critical to success.

With universities under increasing pressure to provide WIL opportunities for greater numbers of students, there is a risk of sacrificing quality for quantity.

Ensuring worthwhile WIL is dependent upon quality supervision, appropriate task allocation and student preparedness, amongst other things. A university student focus group participant indicated that: 'The best placements are when you have something specific to do... not just there to observe something... you have a specific job to do which helps' (Patrick et al., 2009). Bates (2003) adds that the greatest learning occurs in non-theoretical areas and involves the correction of misconceptions about workplace 'reality', and an increased awareness of career options. Participants recognise that WIL should be an integral and integrated part of the curriculum, rather than a 'bolt-on' part of the programme. For example, indicative of the value associated with an integrated approach, several universities are investing efforts in the design and development of a curriculum-wide approach to the development of employability skills from first to final year.

Another major challenge confronting universities is that of providing adequate support for students who undertake work placements. It has long been recognised that the time invested in WIL can be more resource-intensive than the time invested in other modes of learning (Maher & Graves, 2008; Nixon Smith, Stafford, & Camm, 2006). At a practical operational level, questions persist about the extent to which institutions can deliver the flexibility, accessibility and levels of individualisation which are often flagged as positive aspects of WIL. Indeed, Patrick et al. (2009) identify a number of resourcing issues, including workload and time constraints for university and host staff, financial costs to employers and the rigidity of university timetables that can make it difficult to implement strategies. Participants highlight the workload involved in preparing work placements for students. University staff looking for more effective ways to obtain placements for students suggested that new technologies may be part of the solution. One suggestion is the creation of a national database listing universities and faculties seeking placements for students, and industry partners willing to offer work placements. The database could have different portals for different disciplines and work in a similar way to databases used by recruitment agencies (Precision Consultancy, 2007). Effective preparation for effective work placements is seen as much more than just identifying and arranging work placements. Prior to placement, preparation includes planning the pathway through the placement, identifying and managing the diversity of pathways post-placement, and building options and understanding right at the start. The challenges described here must be confronted if Australian universities are to continue to be flexible, adaptive, scholarly and innovative in their approaches to WIL curriculum design and implementation.

10.8 Conclusion

This chapter has highlighted high levels of and distinct expectations on universities in the preparation of students and graduates for the transition to professional practice. These demands are not new. However, the massification of higher education and the switch to user-pays system have increased pressure on universities to find the resources and educational models that will provide relevant, practical experiences that complement more general learning outcomes. Like many other practices, the enactment of WIL is commonly welcomed, albeit for different purposes and with the need to fulfil distinct expectations. There is evidence that learning opportunities connected to the world of work provide a range of benefits for students, including academic, personal, career and work skill development. Drawing on relevant literature and the findings of the national scoping study on WIL, this chapter has provided insights into some of the key tensions existing with the enactment of WIL as a higher education-wide initiative and discussed something of the breadth of activities across the sector and the perceived educational worth of this activity. Fulfilling heightened expectations of industry, students and government will never be easy because, whilst having a common core, there are distinct bases by which students, employers and universities will come to base their judgements about the WIL experience. Consequently, evaluations of this initiative cannot be based on just one of these perspectives (i.e. government, industry, university or students) but through taking measures across these perspectives.

Acknowledgments The authors wish to acknowledge the support provided by the Australian Learning and Teaching Council.

References

Andresen, L., Boud, D., & Cohen, R. (1995). Experience-based learning: Contemporary issues. In G. Foley, (Ed.), *Understanding adult education and training* (2nd ed., pp. 225–239). Sydney, NSW: Allen & Unwin.

Atchison, M., Pollock, S., Reeders, E., & Rizzetti, J. (2002). *Work integrated learning paper.* Melbourne, VIC: Royal Melbourne Institute of Technology.

Australian Learning and Teaching Council. (2010). *The ALTC exchange.* Retrieved March 11, 2010, from http://www.altcexchange.edu.au/

Bates, M. (2003). The assessment of work-integrated learning: Symptoms of personal change. *Journal of Criminal Justice Education, 14*(2), 303–326.

Billett, S. (2001). Knowing in practice: Reconceptualising vocational expertise. *Learning and Instruction, 11*(6), 431–452.

Billett, S. (2009). *Developing agentic professionals through practice-based pedagogies.* [Australian Learning and Teaching Council (ALTC) Fellowship Final Report]. Available online at www.altc.edu.au

Bradley, D., Noonan, P., Nugent, H., & Scales, B. (2008). *Review of Australian higher education: Discussion paper.* Canberra, ACT: Commonwealth of Australia.

Calway, B. (2006). *What has work-integrated learning learned?* Retrieved April 27, 2009, from http://centreforrefs.com/resources/b_calway_2006.pdf

Carapinha, B. (2007, September). *Graduate employability and the European higher education area: An institutional responsibility?* Paper presented at the XIII Annual Assembly CUG, University of Santiago de Compostela, Spain.

Cates, C., Cedercreutz, K. (Eds.) (2008). *Leveraging cooperative education to guide curricular innovation. The development of a corporate feedback system for continuous improvement* (pp. 1–136). Cincinnati, OH: Center for Cooperative Education Research and Innovation: University of Cincinnati.

Consortium for Integrated Resource Management. (2008). *Guidelines for good practice in work integrated learning for the integrated resource sciences.* Prepared for the Consortium for Integrated Resource Management (CIRM). Brisbane, QLD: State of Queensland.

Cooper, L., Orrell, J., & Jones, R. (1999). *Audit of experiential work-based learning programs at Flinders University*. Adelaide, SA: Flinders University.

Davis, R., Franz, J., & Plakalovic, M. (2009). *From WIL to work ready: Evaluating the student-learning continuum, a qualitative study*. Paper presented at the 16th World Association for Cooperative Education (WACE) world conference, Vancouver, Canada.

Department of Education, Employment and Workplace Relations. (2008). *Administrative information for higher education providers: Student support*. Canberra, ACT: Commonwealth of Australia.

Department of Education, Employment and Workplace Relations. (2009). *Transforming Australia's higher education system*. Canberra, ACT: Commonwealth of Australia.

Department of Employment, Education and Training. (1990). *A fair chance for all: National and institutional planning for equity in higher education*. Canberra, ACT: Commonwealth of Australia.

Edwards, D. (2007, September). *Improving student achievement through an industry placement*. Paper presented at the 2007 International Conference on Engineering Education, Coimbra, Portugal.

Fearn, H. (2008, November 27). The class of 2020. *Times Higher Education*, p. 37. http://www.timeshighereducation.co.uk/story.asp?storycode=404431

Gardner, P. (2008). *Ready for prime time? How internships and co-ops affect decisions on full-time job offers*. East Lansing, MI: Michigan State University.

Harvey, L., Moon, S., & Geall, V. (1997). *Graduates work: Organisational change and students' attributes*. Birmingham: Centre for Research into Quality (CRQ) and Association of Graduate Recruiters (AGR).

Knight, P., & Yorke, M. (2004). *Learning, curriculum and employability in higher education*. London: Routledge Falmer.

Kolb, D. (1984). *Experiential learning: Experience as the source of learning and development*. Englewood Cliffs, NJ: Prentice-Hall..

Maher, A., & Graves, S. (2008). *Graduate employability: Can higher education deliver?*. Newbury, Berks: Threshold Press.

Marsick, V. J. (2009). Toward a unifying framework to support informal learning theory, research and practice. *Journal of Workplace Learning, 21*(4), 265–275.

Martin, E. (1997). *The effectiveness of different models of work-based university education* Report prepared for the Department of Employment, Education, Training and Youth Affairs. Canberra, ACT: Commonwealth of Australia.

Martin, E. (1998). Conceptions of workplace university education. *Higher Education Research and Development, 17*(2), 191–205.

McMahon, M., Patton, W., & Tatham, P. (2003). *Managing life learning and work in the 21st century*. Subiaco, WA: Miles Morgan.

Mezirow, J. (1997). Transformative learning: Theory to practice. *New Directions for Adult and Continuing Education, 74*(Summer), 5–12.

Nixon, I., Smith, K., Stafford, R., & Camm, S. (2006). *Work-based learning: Illuminating the higher education landscape*. [The Higher Education Academy (HEA) Final Report]. York: The Higher Education Academy. Available online at: www.heacademy.ac.uk

Orrell, J. (2004). *Work integrated learning programmes: Management and educational quality*. Paper presented at the Australian Universities Quality Forum 2004, Adelaide, Australia. Available online at: http://www.auqa.edu.au/files/publications/auqf2004_proceedings.pdf

O'Shea, A. (2009). *A developmental approach to work integrated learning*. Paper presented at the Australian Collaborative Education Network (ACEN Queensland) September 2009 meeting: Brisbane, Australia.

Patrick, C. -j, Peach, D., Pocknee, C., Webb, F., Fletcher, M., & Pretto, G. (2009). *The WIL [Work Integrated Learning] report: A national scoping study* [Australian Learning and Teaching Council (ALTC) Final Report]. Brisbane: Queensland University of Technology. Available online at: www.altc.edu.au and www.acen.edu.au

Precision Consultancy. (2007). *Graduate employability skills* Prepared for the Business, Industry and Higher Education Collaborative Council. Canberra, ACT: Commonwealth of Australia.

Savage, S. (2005). *Urban Design Education: Learning for Life in Practice* (pp. 3–10). Urban Design International.

Scott, G. (2005). *Accessing the student voice: Using CEQuery to identify what retains students and promotes engagement in productive learning in Australian higher education.* [Department of Education, Science and Training Final Report]. Canberra, ACT: Commonwealth of Australia.

Scott, G. (2008). *University student engagement and satisfaction with learning and teaching.* Sydney, NSW: University of Western Sydney.

Smigiel, H., & Harris, J. (2007). *Audit of work integrated learning programs at Flinders University: A report of the practicum audit.* Adelaide: Flinders University. Available online at: www.flinders.edu.au

Smith, M., Brooks, S., Lichtenberg, A., McIlveen, P., Torjul, P., & Tyler, J. (2009). *Career development learning: Maximising the contribution of work-integrated learning to the student experience.* [Australian Learning and Teaching Council Final Project Report June 2009]. Wollongong: University of Wollongong. Available online at: www.altc.edu.au and www.nagcas.edu.au

Sullivan, W. M., & Rosin, M. S. (2008). *A new agenda for higher education: Shaping a life of the mind for practice.* Indianapolis, IN: Carnegie/Jossey-Bass.

The Panel on Fair Access to the Professions. (2009). *Unleashing aspiration: The final report of the Panel on fair access to the professions.* London: Cabinet Office.

Thurgate, C., & MacGregor, J. (2009). Students' perceptions of undertaking workplace tasks within a foundation degree – health and social care. *Assessment and Evaluation in Higher Education, 34*(2), 149–157.

Universities Australia. (2008). *A national internship scheme: Enhancing the skills and work readiness of Australian university graduates.* Canberra, ACT: Universities Australia.

Chapter 11
Health-Service Organisation, Clinical Team Composition and Student Learning

Maree O'Keefe, Sue McAllister, and Ieva Stupans

11.1 Clinical Work and Learning

Clinical work placements are an integral part of health-profession education programmes. During these placements, students in medicine, dentistry, nursing and allied health join experienced healthcare professionals to work, under skilled supervision, in authentic clinical environments (Dornan, Boshuizen, King, & Scherpbier, 2007; Hilton & Morris, 2001). In doing so, students leave the 'classroom' learning environment of the university and enter the 'real world' of the hospital, dental clinic, community healthcare centre or aged-care facility. This experience is seen as one that provides students with critical support as they transform theory and skills learned in the university context into the ability to practice in the health-service context (Hilton & Morris, 2001).

In contrast to the university setting where education is a primary focus of activity, health services are configured to provide clinical services. Health-service staff often find themselves supervising students in environments where work priorities are centred on patient care rather than on student learning. In such environments, factors such as variable staffing combinations and patient flow arrangements, together with the unpredictability of clinical work, will all significantly influence the learning opportunities available for students. In addition, simultaneously supervising and teaching students while ensuring quality healthcare delivery requires skilful management of multiple roles and responsibilities (Bourbonnais & Kerr, 2007; Carlisle, Cooper, & Watkins, 2004; McCormack & Slater, 2006).

Health services are complex and dynamic learning environments where the patient or client rather than the student is the primary focus of activity and where opportunities to learn through participation may vary (Le Maistre & Pare, 2004; Lyon, 2004). Yet, for students, health workplaces are often unique learning environments in which they can be legitimate, albeit peripheral, participants (Lave

M. O'Keefe (✉)
University of Adelaide, Adelaide, SA, Australia
e-mail: maree.okeefe@adelaide.edu.au

S. Billett, A. Henderson (eds.), *Developing Learning Professionals*, Professional
and Practice-based Learning 7, DOI 10.1007/978-90-481-3937-8_11,
© Springer Science+Business Media B.V. 2011

& Wenger, 1991). Indeed, the quality of the student-learning experience in clinical placements is often reflected at least in part by the extent to which students can participate as legitimate 'worker-learners' (Boor et al., 2008; Dornan et al., 2007). Unsurprisingly, therefore, when students are not viewed as legitimate participants in clinical environments, they are more likely to disengage from active learning (Boor et al., 2008).

It follows then that in considering the nature of student-learning opportunities in clinical placements, the following questions can be posed:

a. How do differing clinical team compositions and work responsibilities shape student-learning opportunities?
b. How do clinical team members negotiate responsibility for student-learning outcomes within their team?
c. How do health-service organisational structures impact on the opportunities clinical teams have to work together to ensure high-quality student-learning experiences?

These questions are explored further throughout this chapter drawing on three examples of student clinical placements in health-service settings. The distribution of clinical teaching activities within multidisciplinary teams is considered against the need in these clinical settings to balance patient and client service responsibilities and teaching. Opportunities for clinical teams to negotiate responsibility for student learning are discussed together with factors influencing clinical team responsiveness to students' learning needs. It is argued that workload pressures and variable clinical team composition reinforce a strongly discipline-based approach to managing student supervision, and that health-service organisation significantly influences the ways in which clinical team members can plan and support student learning.

11.2 Discipline Identities and Responsibilities Within Clinical Teams

Although healthcare providers use a variety of service delivery models, common to the organisation of each service is some form of teamwork. Within individual healthcare services, the composition of clinical teams (for example, the surgeons, anaesthetists and nursing staff who work together regularly in operating theatres) and the responsibilities of individual members can be fairly stable over time. In other situations, such as in the management of acutely ill or injured patients, the type of healthcare being provided will determine the composition of clinical teams, the time the team works together and the responsibilities of individual team members (Flin & Maran, 2004; Manser, 2009). One example where different combinations of healthcare workers come together in acute care situations according to the specific needs of different patients is in hospital emergency departments. In addition, even within stable work teams, fluidity in the composition of team membership on any day can be introduced by factors such as shift work, the use of part-time work and backfill temporary and casual staff. Individual staff members may also be members of more than one team for different work functions, and may move between teams to flexibly respond to patient-care workload demands.

Within health-service teams, the clinical workload is often shared among team members according to (i) patient and client healthcare needs, (ii) individual team member expertise and experience, (iii) the distribution and balance of workload across team members, and (iv) the service delivery model and philosophy of the healthcare organisation. There are, however, recognised limits to the extent to which workload can be shared across different disciplines (Catchpole, Mishra, Handa, & McCulloch, 2008; Manser, Harrison, Gaba, & Howard, 2009). Although many healthcare teams have multidisciplinary membership, typically workload distribution occurs according to recognised disciplinary groupings within each team. Distinct discipline identities within clinical teams are often further reinforced by professional development activities that clarify or make explicit distinct staff roles in emergency and other high-stress situations, so as to improve patient-care quality and safety outcomes (Flin & Maran, 2004).

Disciplinary distinctions within clinical teams are also seen in the organisation of students' clinical placements. There is often an implicit assumption by university staff and external professional accreditation agencies that, during their clinical placements, students will predominantly work with, and be the responsibility of, those member(s) of the clinical team who are of the same discipline as the student. As a result, university staff who organise and coordinate student clinical placements tend to liaise only with representatives of the same discipline within each health service. Although there are obvious efficiencies with such a discipline-focused process of student-learning support, the fact that the students interact with, and can learn from, an entire clinical team during their placement is sometimes overlooked. Therefore, in order to understand how placement organisation and coordination can best play out across clinical settings, it is necessary to investigate some instances of practice. These learnings can then be used to guide practices in clinical settings.

11.3 Three Examples of Clinical Placements in Health-Service Teams

As part of a project to identify and build leadership capacity for quality student learning within clinical teams, a model for team development was tested in three different health-service teams.[1] As part of this project, members of participating

[1] These three clinical teams participated in the Leadership for Excellence Project 'Using TMS to identify and build leadership for quality learning in clinical healthcare teams.' Support for the project was provided by the Australian Learning and Teaching Council, an initiative of the Australian Government Department of Education, Employment and Workplace Relations. The

clinical teams investigated the extent to which they could work individually and/or collectively to improve student-learning opportunities within their team.

The project involved sequential engagement with clinical teams with increasingly complex organisational and coordination structures in terms of the following: (a) *team composition*: the number and range of different disciplines represented within the team; (b) *student programmes*: the number of different discipline programmes placing students with the team; and (c) *university relationships*: the number of universities placing students within the team.

Through creating different combinations of these criteria, three contrasting and increasingly complex clinical team profiles were constructed:

- Team 1: a single health-profession team with students from one health-profession programme and one university
- Team 2: a multidisciplinary health-profession team with students from one or two health-profession programmes and one or two universities
- Team 3: a rural, multidisciplinary health-profession team with students from more than one health-profession programme and three universities

Three clinical teams were identified, each from a different health service, to match these profiles. Baseline data regarding team membership and student clinical placements were gathered through interviews and field observations. Participating team members completed two profiling activities and associated workshops in which they identified their personal work preferences when supporting students' learning, and evaluated their own team's performance as a learning environment. The following three teams participated in the project.

- Team 1: A single profession team with students from one health-profession programme and one university

    - The team: The first team was situated in a community dental service that was part of a large state-wide organisation providing a range of public dental services. The service was relatively self-contained and most of the dental service team staff participated in the project. The dental clinic operated on an appointment basis, 5 days per week. Participating team members included three dentists (one of whom was the clinical leader), one dental therapist, two dental assistants and one practice manager.
    - The students: Students from one university, who were studying to be dentists, were placed with this dental service during their final year of study. A series of 2-week placements occurred throughout the year with two students attending at one time. During the placement, students provided dental treatment to patients under the supervision of one of the dentists. The dental assistants worked with the students in the same way they worked with the dentists when

views expressed in this publication do not necessarily reflect the views of the Australian Learning and Teaching Council or of the Australian Government.

providing patient care. Student supervision was shared by formal arrangement between the dentists. The clinical leader undertook most of the supervision and workload adjustments were in place in recognition of these extra duties.

- Team 2: A multidisciplinary health-profession team with students from one or two health-profession programmes and one or two universities

  - The team: The second team was situated in a residential aged-care facility that was part of a large service providing home- and community-based services to support the aged. Client care was provided on a 24-h basis by a number of clinical teams that differed in composition from day to day. As a result of different individual team member work schedules (i.e. due to shift and part-time work), members of these different clinical teams rarely met as an entire group. While there was some stability in the membership of different care teams within the aged-care facility, all members of any one particular care team could not be simultaneously available to participate in project activities unlike in the dental clinic. Therefore, a representative group of staff from across the facility was sought for the project to form a 'team' for the purposes of the project. Participating health-service staff included the nurse manager, a volunteer/activities coordinator, a visiting physiotherapist, two registered nurses, two enrolled nurses and two aged-care workers.
  - The students: Nursing, aged-care, physiotherapy and pharmacy students were placed with the facility for variable lengths of time depending on their programme of study and institution (i.e. two universities and several technical and further education institutions placed students with this service). Nursing student placements only were available to be observed during the project period. During their clinical placements nursing students were rostered to attend the aged-care facility for either day or evening work shifts. The nurse manager determined the allocation of individual students across the facility according to the overall learning objectives stipulated by their higher education institution, and according to the student's progress within their study programme. Subsequently, the registered nurse in charge of the shift oversaw the allocation of specific tasks and activities to the student for that shift. This allocation was influenced in part by the registered nurse's understanding of the student's learning objectives and the learning opportunities available through the shift, and in part by the number and kinds of tasks to be completed during the shift. While the registered nurse had overall responsibility for student supervision, some responsibility was devolved to other members of the clinical team (for example, the enrolled nurse) depending on the tasks being undertaken.

- Team 3: A rural, multidisciplinary health-profession team with students from more than one health-profession programme and three universities

  - The team: The third team was situated in a country hospital where both acute and long-term patient care were provided 24 h a day. Services at the hospital were provided by a number of clinical teams comprising onsite staff (i.e. nurses, administrative staff and other service personnel), and doctors who worked in a community-based general practice as well as at the hospital. As with the aged-care facility at which the second team was based, it was not possible to simply enrol one of these clinical teams to participate in the project because of their ongoing obligation to provide continuous healthcare for patients. Therefore, as was the case in the aged-care facility, a representative group of staff was selected. Participating country hospital staff included two doctors, two registered nurses, an enrolled nurse, a midwife, a student coordinator and a ward clerk.

– The students: Clinical placements within the hospital were provided for medical students from two universities and nursing students from three universities. Diversity in the range of education programmes, placement organisation by discipline, student prior experience and knowledge, and each university's expectations for student learning were more marked than in either the dental or aged-care teams. Medical students were allocated to the external medical practice where they worked alongside the doctors who provided supervision. These medical students visited the hospital with the doctors for specific patient care as required. Nursing students were rostered onto the wards in work shifts in the same manner as nursing students at the aged-care facility. These nursing students assisted with general nursing care under the supervision of the registered nurse in charge of that shift. As with the aged-care facility, tasks and activities were allocated to the student in part according to the registered nurse's understanding of the student's learning objectives and assessment requirements, and in part according to the workload.

11.4 Balancing Service and Teaching

The project outcomes supported the earlier proposed view that, in health services, workload pressures and the variable nature of clinical team composition would likely reinforce a primarily discipline-based approach to managing student learning. This outcome was observed despite the multidisciplinary composition of the clinical work teams participating in the project. In addition, health-service organisation was an important additional factor in determining the ways in which clinical team members could plan and support students' learning. The more complex the health-service organisation, in terms of variability in clinical team composition, patient and client care responsibilities and the overall size of the organisation, the fewer opportunities staff had to meet as a team to discuss student learning. Further complicating this picture was the fact that the more complex the health service, especially in terms of size, the greater the number of universities placing students and the greater the number of different programmes and levels of study represented, rendering the task of planning more difficult.

In addition to student supervision and teaching, each health service was responsible for the maintenance of appropriate health-service levels and quality. For the three clinical teams, the number and type of learning opportunities that could be made available to students was heavily dependent on concurrent healthcare service responsibilities (i.e. when a clinical team had a high service workload, the number and range of student-learning opportunities decreased). The effect of service responsibilities on learning and teaching practices within the service environment differed across the three teams, as did each team member's perceptions of and/or responses to difficulties that arose in trying to balance service and teaching responsibilities. In many instances, teaching and supervising students was seen as competing with patient care.

For the dental clinic staff, while the students' role in assisting service provision was valued, there was on-going concern among members of the staff about their ability to simultaneously manage patient caseloads and keep waiting lists from becoming too long, while also teaching and supervising their students. The different level of individual dental students' clinical skill contributed to these concerns. During their clinical placements, some students demonstrated high levels of proficiency in dental care and could work as quickly as the dentists with minimal supervisor intervention. Yet, students who were not as experienced or as competent required much longer than a standard appointment time to complete some patient treatments. In this situation, students often also required considerable assistance from the supervisor and, consequently, patient waiting times increased. Complicating matters further, each student had a unique profile of experience and competence and, therefore, required different amounts of additional time from supervisors depending on the treatment needs of the patients. This unpredictability in the time each student needed to treat any one patient created major scheduling difficulties for the dental practice manager who tried to keep patient waiting times to a minimum. It was particularly frustrating for the practice manager that information on individual student proficiency was not available prior to the commencement of each clinical placement. As a result, the practice manager was constantly reviewing and revising patient appointment times on the student's patient lists to ensure service delivery standards were maintained.

Members of both the aged-care and country hospital teams also described difficulties associated with balancing student learning while simultaneously delivering appropriate levels of client and patient care. These difficulties were compounded by a range of factors including variability in (i) clinical placement length and timing across year levels and disciplines; (ii) university administrative practices; (iii) the nature of each student's learning objectives and assessment tasks; and (iv) the requirements for supervision and assessment for each staff member. The management of student learning became more difficult as the number of educational institutions placing students at any one time, the numbers of different programmes placing students, and the range of different skill levels of students all increased.

The variety of, and at times mismatch between, educational institutions' requirements for student learning and the context of service delivery at times contributed to confusion and concern on the part of the staff for the quality of the student experience. Members in each of the participating teams in the project were aware of and tried to respond to challenges associated with the simultaneous delivery of quality healthcare while still meeting student-learning expectations and needs. Many intentions on the part of the clinical staff however well intentioned were unable to be realised, especially in relation to preparation and planning for student placements. When clinical staff tried to plan ahead to better manage student learning within their existing workloads, these efforts were often thwarted because information about students' learning needs was unavailable prior to them commencing their placement. When this occurred, students were at greater risk of not achieving their desired learning outcomes (Wray & McCall, 2009). In all, and not surprisingly, the greater the number of institutions and programmes placing students with a health service, the greater the problem of inadequate communication between clinical team members and university staff became. From these scenarios can be seen the need to recognise that the development of a future health workforce is a shared responsibility of both universities and health services (Rodger et al., 2008). Also rehearsing what had been found previously, it is evident that formal support for clinical teams from health services and/or universities is important to help clinical team members manage students' learning (Bourbonnais & Kerr, 2007; Carlisle et al., 2004; McCormack & Slater, 2006). That is, even with the best and most professional of intentions the compounding factors of multiple students with different levels of clinical competence and readiness to practice, all of which is unknowable until the students commence their placement, suggest that clinicians' planning to assist student learning is unlikely to be successful.

Student supervision was, not surprisingly, perceived as adding to the workload of health-service staff. Although staff enjoyed their teaching roles most of the time, the tension between teaching and managing their workload was often professionally frustrating for the clinicians. Team members viewed students as potential future colleagues and were acutely aware of the potential relationship between the quality of the student placement experience and future staff recruitment outcomes. Moreover, they hoped that positive learning experiences would encourage students to return and work in the service once they had graduated. Given the difficulties faced by clinicians, it is necessary to understand the premises upon which universities organise and provide placements for their students.

11.5 Health-Service Organisation and Clinical Team Responsiveness to Student-Learning Needs

Considerable variability was found across higher education institutions in their requirements of health services for clinical placements. In addition to different learning objectives and assessment practices, each university had distinct processes for managing student placements and health-service liaison. Overlaying this diversity in higher education practices, the diversity in health-service organisation further complicated the management of student clinical placements for clinical team members. Working through the process of identifying and enrolling each of the participating teams for the project permitted some observations to be made by members of the project team about the ways in which health-service organisation shaped students' learning opportunities. In particular, health-service organisation was seen to be an important factor in determining the ways in which clinical team members came together to plan and support student learning. Health-service organisation was important also in determining the extent to which students could become legitimate participants in the provision of healthcare, both in the extent to which the workplace was supportive of student learning (Dornan et al., 2007) and in the relationships between team members and students (Boor et al., 2008; Lyon, 2004). Within the three teams participating in the project, all members were individually supportive of, and committed to, high-quality student-learning experiences. The extent to which each clinical team could realise this aspiration was, however, determined to a large extent by organisational factors that were beyond the team's control.

When compared with the dental clinic, the more complex organisational environments of the aged-care facility and the country hospital allowed much less flexibility for clinical staff to negotiate any modifications to their daily activities. Aged-care and country hospital team members also had few opportunities to support each other in their teaching roles because of their continuous patient-care responsibilities and the changing composition of clinical work teams as discussed above. In contrast, in the relatively stable dental team, team members met regularly as a group to discuss clinical matters. This resulted in greater capacity among members of the dental clinical team to reorganise the way in which student learning was integrated into service delivery.[2]

In both the aged-care facility and the country hospital, students came from multiple institutions and programmes and with a range of clinical competency levels. These factors added to the complexity arising from patient-care responsibilities and changing team composition. The educational institutions placing the students provided different amounts and types of information regarding their students' learning needs and assessment requirements. A further complication for both the aged-care facility and the country hospital teams was the fact that most communication between the universities and the respective health services was managed administratively in a part of the organisation that was remote from the staff who were supervising the students and without any direct involvement with them. With little opportunity for planning, busy clinical staff often had no option other than to respond in an ad hoc manner to students' learning and assessment needs.

It was also apparent that, for all three teams, having to manage staff turnover and staff absences due to ill health together with the coordination of part-time worker schedules had a significant impact on the nature of learning experiences available to students. For example, in the dental clinic, if a dental assistant was absent, one dental student patient list would be cancelled so that one of the students could act as dental assistant for the other student. Shift work rosters also created some discontinuity in

---

[2]Despite having less autonomy to reorganise their day-to-day activities to improve student learning opportunities, as a result of participation in the project, both the aged-care and country hospital teams identified and created changes within their organisations to enhance student learning.

student supervision by staff, because this broke the continuity of the engagement across the team.

For each of the teams, service organisation structures and clinical workload were key factors in determining whether clinical team members could meet to discuss learning and teaching; to plan, implement and monitor innovations and quality improvements in student-learning opportunities; and to share and support each other in providing this learning. So, these arrangements affected not only the ability of clinical team members to assist students, but also many other facets of their work. However, as the priority was for patient care, complicated student support arrangements increased the tendency for student learning to become a peripheral consideration for clinical staff. These same factors (i.e. service organisation structures and clinical workload) could also disrupt learning relationships between individual staff and students. Through the project, however, it was seen that each of the teams could be supported to identify opportunities to work within these constraints to create and maintain positive learning environments for their students. This is now discussed as a process of negotiating responsibility.

11.6 Negotiating Responsibility for Student Learning Within Clinical Teams

From the beginning, the project team adopted a pedagogical viewpoint that students could learn about clinical practice from all members of the clinical team, not just members of their own discipline during their placement. However, it became apparent during the project that while clinical team members were clear about their work roles, their understanding of the range of possible teaching roles they could play differed widely. This conclusion is consistent with previous observations that members of healthcare teams differ in their perceptions of the performance of other team members from different disciplines (Manser, 2009). Participating team members in this project had greater confidence in their discipline-specific roles in supporting student learning than in their ability to support the more generic aspects of student learning. This outcome is probably not surprising given the imperatives of healthcare delivery where greater quality is associated with greater role clarification within teams and less distribution of roles among team members (Manser et al., 2009; Flin & Maran, 2004).

The extent to which team members undertook any negotiation among themselves about addressing student-learning needs declined as the complexity of health-service organisation and clinical placement arrangements increased. In more complex situations, such as clinical teams where there was daily changing membership, with students from different disciplines and universities and with different level of competencies, team members had few, if any, opportunities to support each other in their teaching roles.

Negotiation of responsibility for student learning was again more straightforward in less complex situations. The dental team members who participated in the project were all members of a well-defined team that existed prior to the project. It was observed that there were clear roles relating to patient care for every team member including the dental students. As an established clinical team, members had a range of existing communication mechanisms within the group to discuss matters relating to their clinical practice. These mechanisms were also used to negotiate the management of student learning. The same established mechanisms gave students the opportunity to give feedback on their learning experiences. Most importantly, although the dentists were responsible for the teaching and supervision of students, every member of the team knew why the student was placed with their service and what the students' learning objectives were. The dental students may have been primarily the responsibility of the dentists. Yet, as the project unfolded, a wider range of team members, in addition to the dentist, were able to articulate a role for themselves in supporting student learning. Students were given a greater number of opportunities to customise their learning experiences, including the opportunity to request certain types of clinical work and consultation times.

Although the participating aged-care team members all worked at the same aged-care service, participants in this project did not usually work together as a single stable team. On a daily basis, and depending on which other staff were rostered to work in different work shifts, the aged-care team members would take on slightly different work responsibilities. Team members also needed to readjust to their precise clinical roles for each shift based on the current workload. This process of negotiation of clinical workload according to team composition and required task for each shift made it much more difficult to determine who had the key responsibility for ensuring that students were achieving their learning objectives; and team members had a less detailed understanding of their students' learning needs than was seen, for example, in the dental team.

A different situation again was observed in the country hospital team. Unlike the other two clinical teams participating in the project, as the project progressed, there emerged two subgroups of clinical staff within the country hospital clinical team. The first subgroup included staff such as the nurses and the ward clerk who worked shifts in the hospital and who were responsible for both nursing and medical students. The second subgroup included the doctors who worked primarily in their medical practice, visiting the hospital as required for patient care. These doctors were responsible for medical students only. While the doctors had a good understanding of their individual roles and the medical students' learning objectives across several year levels, the hospital staff had a much less clear understanding of the learning objectives of the students placed with them (i.e. both nursing and medical students). For the nurses also, the precise nature of their clinical roles varied across work shifts depending on the composition of the team for that shift. In addition, as with the aged-care team, although the participating clinical team members all worked together at the same service, they rarely if ever came together at work as a single team. Making these arrangements even more difficult for the hospital staff was the fact that the students placed with this country hospital came from a range of different universities, programmes and levels of study.

In the country hospital team, management of student learning was seen to be organised along disciplinary lines and there was little communication between different discipline groups in any forum, especially between nurses and doctors, and between nursing students and medical students.[3] While medical students were always supernumerary learners, in some instances nursing students were simultaneously both workers and learners. The extent to which clinical team members were able to negotiate responsibility for student learning was related to a number of factors, including the complexity of the health service and the clinical team's workload. A lack of clarity around the key learning objectives guiding student learning further impeded the development of a team approach to managing student learning. Stronger partnerships between health services and universities would likely provide clinical teams with greater support as they manage student learning on a day-to-day basis.

11.7 Strengthening Health Service and University Partnerships for Student Learning

At the beginning of this chapter, three questions were posed in relation to health professional student-learning opportunities and experiences in health-service clinical placements. These questions related to the impact of (a) clinical team composition and workload; (b) the extent to which responsibility for student-learning outcomes was or could be negotiated; and (c) health-service organisation.

In the three teams participating in the project, there was a distinct disciplinary framework that linked the type of health-profession students who were placed, with clinical team composition and the student-learning activities that were available to them. Nursing students primarily learned from nurses, dental students from dentists and so on. Where more than one discipline was represented within the clinical team, as in the country hospital team, student supervision primarily rested with the members of the team who belonged to the same discipline. Such strong disciplinary linkages and expectations were associated with some potential interdisciplinary learning opportunities being overlooked, or 'falling between the cracks'. Workload pressures and the variable composition of some teams on a day-to-day basis served to reinforce a model of a mono-disciplinary approach to student learning. Such a model was widely perceived by clinical staff as the only one with which staff could cope while still meeting their clinical service requirements.

There were limited opportunities for clinical teams to meet as a team to discuss a range of matters about their practice, one of which was student learning. As a result, clinical team members often assumed responsibility for student learning individually in an uncoordinated fashion. The project was successful in providing clinical team members with the opportunity to reflect on their roles as teachers, and

---

[3]The country hospital team was the only one of the three teams in which students from more than one discipline were observed in the same workplace.

recognise their collective ability to plan and implement teaching improvements that would not compromise clinical service delivery.

The insights gained through this project also suggest that there is a need for university staff to develop a greater understanding of health-service organisation and how this impacts on students' learning experiences. In particular, there should be a good understanding of the nature of teamwork within each individual health service, together with the full range of opportunities available for students to participate in clinical practice. Appreciating the specific nature of teamwork within a health service may lead university staff in some instances to consider working with 'team' rather than with individual discipline contacts. University staff should also be aware that information flow about students' learning objectives might differ within and across organisations. It is likely that a range of tailored strategies is needed to ensure supervising clinical staff have access to specific information on student-learning objectives and assessment requirements.

From the perspective of health services, the project outcomes suggest that there is a need to create time for clinical team members to meet and discuss their teaching roles and responsibilities. Ways in which work can be structured to more effectively meet both service priorities and student-learning needs could then be explored and opportunities to share this work across team members identified. Coupled with these team-based activities, health services might consider strategies for effective communication throughout their organisation to assist in disseminating information about student learning.

As noted earlier, as well as considerations about the experiences afforded to students, consideration should also be given to the way students perceive themselves to be engaged in clinical work. If students feel that they are peripheral to the daily activities of the clinical team, they are likely to not engage richly and effortfully. So, beyond what clinicians do or do not do, students' engagement in their learning will be influenced by how they believe they are being permitted to participate. Clearly a one-size-fits-all approach is not going to work for either the clinicians or the students – but much good will exists within health services at all levels to partner with universities to improve the integration of service and teaching. What is required are negotiations across institutions that are sensitive to the complexities of the practice and also mindful of the need for students to be supported and engaged in ways that allow them to contribute and learn effectively in doing so.

Acknowledgments We acknowledge the contribution of the clinical teams and health services who participated in this project together with the Building Leadership for Quality Learning project team. We also acknowledge the support provided by the Australian Learning and Teaching Council.

References

Boor, K., Scheele, F., van der Vleuten, C. P. M., Teunissen, P. W., den Breejen, E. M. E., & Scherpbier, A. J. J. A. (2008). How undergraduate clinical learning climates differ: A multi-method case study. *Medical Education, 42*(7), 1029–1036.

Bourbonnais, F. F., & Kerr, E. (2007). Preceptoring a student in the final clinical placement: Reflections from nurses in a Canadian hospital. *Journal of Clinical Nursing, 16*(8), 1543–1547.

Carlisle, C., Cooper, H., & Watkins, C. (2004). Do none of you talk to each other?: The challenges facing the implementation of inter-professional education. *Medical Teacher, 26*(6), 545–552.

Catchpole, K., Mishra, A., Handa, A., & McCulloch, P. (2008). Teamwork and error in the operating room. Analysis of skills and roles. *Annals of Surgery, 247*(4), 699–706.

Dornan, T., Boshuizen, H., King, N., & Scherpbier, A. (2007). Experience-based learning: A model linking the processes and outcomes of medical students' workplace learning. *Medical Education, 41*(1), 84–91.

Flin, R., & Maran, N. (2004). Identifying and training non-technical skills for teams in acute medicine. *Quality and Safety in Health Care, 13*(suppl. 1), i80–i84. DOI:10.1136/qshc.2004.009993.

Hilton, R., & Morris, J. (2001). Student placements- Is there evidence supporting team skills development in clinical practice settings?. *Journal of Interprofessional Care, 15*(2), 171–183.

Lave, J., & Wenger, E. (1991). *Situated learning: Legitimate peripheral participation.* New York: Cambridge University Press.

Le Maistre, C., & Pare, A. (2004). Learning in two communities: The challenge for universities and workplaces. *Journal of Workplace Learning, 16*(1/2), 44–52.

Lyon, P. (2004). A model of teaching and learning in the operating theatre. *Medical Education, 38*(12), 1278–1287.

Manser, T. (2009). Teamwork and patient safety in dynamic domains of healthcare: A review of the literature. *Acta Anaesthesiology Scandanavia, 53*(2), 143–151.

Manser, T., Harrison, T. K., Gaba, D. M., & Howard, S. K. (2009). Coordination pattern related to high clinical performance in a simulated anesthetic crisis. *Anesthetic Analgesia, 108*(5), 1606–1615.

McCormack, B., & Slater, P. (2006). An evaluation of the clinical education facilitator. *Journal of Clinical Nursing, 15*(2), 135–144.

Rodger, S., Webb, G., Devitt, L., Gilbert, J., Wrightson, P., & McMeekin, J. (2008). Clinical education and practice placements in the allied health professions: An international perspective. *Journal of Allied Health, 37*(1), 53–62.

Wray, N., & McCall, L. (2009). 'They don't know much about us': Educational reform impacts on students' learning in the clinical environment. *Advances in Health Sciences Education, 14*(5), 665–676.

Chapter 12
Promoting Professional Learning: Individual and Institutional Practices and Imperatives

Amanda Henderson

12.1 Assisting the Effective Integration of Experiences in University and Practice Settings

Providing access to real-world experiences for students is imperative to introduce them to how knowledge can inform practice and also for them to explore how engagement in authentic practice can contribute to the meanings that they formulate initially as students, and then later throughout their professional working life. Yet, shaping student learning within authentic health and human service settings to assist this learning is a challenge given the unpredictable nature of the situations that can present and how students respond and learn from and through these circumstances. In this way, the unpredictability of learning and meanings derived are further complicated by the experiences that individual students bring to the practice situation and which shape how they construct their knowledge. The range of scenarios, situational learning and case studies presented across the chapters in this book emphasise the importance for authentic institutional experiences through the opportunity for students to integrate canonical, situational and personal manifestations because, as previously noted (see Chapter 2, this volume), they are interconnected and interdependent. The difficulty in structuring learning experiences is how this complex of considerations plays out so that the authentic nature of situations that the student experiences can be directed towards the student securing a level of initial professional preparation that will permit them to work effectively as a healthcare professional. Preparation for this entry level of practice means that the student should be able to attend to their clients' needs upon graduation; though it is acknowledged that their practice is 'under supervision' at this stage. Yet, they still require a level of personal competence because depending on the workplace arrangements this supervision can be direct or indirect.

Of particular interest in the structuring of learning experiences for students is the development of knowledge beyond the canonical; that is, an understanding of the

A. Henderson (✉)
Queensland Health, Queensland, Australia; School of Nursing and Midwifery, Griffith University, Queensland, Australia
e-mail: Amanda_Henderson@health.qld.gov.au

human condition when experiencing health deviations, based on situational aspects and the personally constructed domain of occupational knowledge. The importance of practice-based settings is the opportunity for individuals to construct this knowledge, as it cannot be taught; rather, it needs to be learnt (see Chapter 2, this volume). Exposure to 'real-life' situations, therefore, is the catalyst for students to develop this contextual knowledge. In the process of promoting learning within human services and clinical healthcare settings, tensions between individual understanding of professional practice and preferences on the one hand, and institutional imperatives on the other, can become apparent and in ways that can subvert the intended learning outcomes.

The creation of ideal learning scenarios can assist learners move towards the effective integration of knowledge, understanding and experiences so that the performance of professional practice becomes more coherent to the student and results in embedding knowledge and practice that subsequently provides good outcomes for clients. This learning directly aids the development of professional judgement. Professional judgement expertise is a core component of learning across professional practice – it is one of the five core learning outcomes recognised by the Dublin Descriptors (Joint Quality Initiative informal group, 2004). It is not purely students' extensive exposure to or observed experience of situations that lend themselves to the development of sound judgement. Instead, the engagement of learners also is mandatory so that assimilation of knowledge and reflections from the experiences can be assured (see Chapter 2, this volume).

Of consideration here, however, is that actual practice is fluid. That is, it cannot be predicted with any certainty. Preparation for the practice environment, and support within this environment, is, therefore, essential to cater for this uncertainty. Students need to be knowledgeable about the broad contexts of human services and healthcare practices and situations that staff need to manage, in order to be able to respond effectively to emerging challenges and complex healthcare requirements. Furthermore, students need to be equipped with 'survival skills' to deal with the diversity of situations in which they may find themselves. For instance, many students may experience dissonance between what ought to happen and what actually happens in healthcare settings. In the absence of a definitive curricula structure that assures student success in acquiring the broad range of practice abilities that lead them to make sense of their experiences and ultimately deliver sound judgements, the different healthcare professions approach practice preparation within the curricula in many different ways. Therefore, it is necessary to propose some ways in which this unpredictable and uncertain process can be organised to shape as best as possible learning through practice.

12.2 Staging and Sequencing of Learning in Practice

Depending on the curricula of a particular discipline or institution, students can be provided with minimal guidelines and support for exploring how they may contribute to the healthcare provisions during their clinical practicum. These practicums can occur when students are nearing completion of their qualification, and may require the student to demonstrate sound judgement in very specific tasks and activities in order to complete their degree. Alternatively, students' exposure to clinical practice can be a staged approach where criteria for engagement can be sequenced through an ordered hierarchy of skills. A number of perspectives have been presented throughout the chapters in this book (from disciplines such as physiotherapy, midwifery, medicine, nursing and human services) about students' imperatives for learning, the relationship of these with institutional imperatives, and how structuring and support for these experiences can facilitate learning that culminates in the student being able to effectively reason about clinical problems. Even though challenges and contexts appear quite diverse, there are key factors that emerge as important for practice-based learning. Consideration of these key factors is worthwhile if the opportunities afforded from workplace learning are to be effectively optimised.

A value of structuring learning experiences within the clinical practicum is the potential for focused and deliberate practice (Ericson, 2006). For physiotherapy, midwifery, medicine and nursing students, the instructions about the intent of the practice situation were premised on skills and attributes recognised as central to students' needs upon graduation. How learning around these central skills and attributes progressed, however, was a rather broad interpretation of the intended curriculum. In particular, the learning around the requisite activities appeared to be based on preconceived ideas of what students believed was important for them to know. The deliberate practice as established by the academic institution was not adopted in its entirety by the learner – rather, the deliberate practice actively sought by the learner was often more specific. The limitation of students' ideas about what was important for them to know was largely based on their preconceived and potentially limited understanding of the scope of their professional work. That is, their experiences to date shaped the scope and direction of their intentional learning. Arguably, students can be naive about the exact nature of their work and, therefore, what is fundamental for them to perform their professional work. These preconceived notions can be strong in influencing how the students approach their work and ultimately what they will learn as a consequence of that work.

When students are placed in the work setting, their ideas about practice are formulated through their 'lens' – that is, what they believe is the intent of their practice. This lens directly influences how the students make sense of the continuous information that is afforded to them both directly and indirectly during practice situations. Through the lens, arguably their preconceived ideas, and then the filter that will assist them make sense of these ideas, students come to understand their professional practice. The lens and filter will ultimately shape how they create meaning through their activities and their learning. Optimum preparation of students involves opening the lens as widely as possible and managing the nature of the filter to ensure essential learning experiences are captured.

The case studies presented from the areas of physiotherapy, midwifery and interprofessional learning opportunities highlighted the tensions between student intentions around their learning and the proposed learning objectives of the curricula based on the educational institutions' desired outcomes. It became apparent, particularly in the profession of physiotherapy, that students prioritised tasks and these were different from the tasks prioritised by the educational institutions.

12.3 Student Priorities in Learning

The short week-long programme designed by Molloy and Keating (see Chapter 4, p. x, this volume) was intended 'to make transparent the expectations of clinical education' and, arguably of greater importance, 'to provide students with further knowledge and skills in self-directed learning as a means of negotiating the complexity and uncertainty of the clinical environment.' However, students have strong intentionality that directs their learning. Students demonstrated a strong preoccupation with the acquisition and ability to perform technical/procedural skills. Molloy and Keating summarised from their short programme designed to better prepare students for their clinical experience that students viewed the professional aspects of their physiotherapy role as 'peripheral' to their core business. These reflections were based on feedback from the students after participation in the week-long preparation for clinical practice, however, before the students commenced the clinical experience component of their learning.

The need to equip students with professional behaviours and techniques for learning in complex situations would seem to be mandatory given that the workloads in the clinical environments in which students are placed are often heavy and demanding (Rodgers et al., 2008). Healthcare students need the professional skills to seek and negotiate learning opportunities with staff as they become available, as staff are not always adequately prepared to structure the learning experience for students (Brammer, 2006). The demands of clinical settings mean that, unlike university situations where students are invited to participate, and often have time for preparation and reflection around the requisite skills that are being practised, diverse learning opportunities can emerge spontaneously. In these circumstances, students are not afforded the benefits of time for a preparation prior to engaging in a practice situation. Therefore, preparation of the students to both recognise and utilise the opportunities afforded is needed prior to placement experiences. Professional skills such as communication and collaboration with both the client and the team can directly assist the student to engage, learn and reflect.

Molloy and Keating (Chapter 4, this volume) acknowledge that students' focus on skill acquisition may be influenced by a survival approach adopted by the students for the first clinical practicum. Maybe if students can 'do,' then, ultimately, they may derive confidence in the professional interactions that are common and fundamental to their practice. While physiotherapy students may initially understand their profession in a predominantly biomedical sense – and this may be appropriate if they are to develop the precision skills in manipulation of the body to bring about the desired outcomes – the complexity of physiotherapy work may emerge subsequent to the refinement of their 'hands on' skills.

This priority for students to adopt a largely task-focused approach did not dominate the preparation only of the physiotherapy students during their preparation for clinical practicum. Instead, the focus on tasks dominated the learning priorities of students of other professional groups during the clinical experiences. Of particular interest for understanding students' development is that often different approaches to learning designed to expand students' 'tool set' were not perceived as important by students. The students' 'tool set' is the repertoire of tasks that they need to be able to perform to appear credible within the work context in which they are situated.

The different approach to learning as structured by the 'follow through experience' during the midwifery programme (described in Chapter 5, this volume) is just one example. The intent of the follow-through experience in the midwifery programme was for midwives to follow a pregnant woman through from pregnancy to birth. As Glover and Sweet explain, in the development of the Bachelor of Midwifery, academic staff formulated a definition of the follow through; however, the definition offered few insights into the actual practice of how students were to engage in learning around the follow-through experience. The follow-through experience lacked clarity and, therefore, its outcomes as they pertained to student learning were variable. As already noted, learning in context, whether highly structured or flexible, is largely subject to students' perceptions about professional work. The approach adopted in this programme initially involved observation by the students, which eventually, depending on the circumstances, involved participation of the student in the midwifery care of the birthing woman. Creating the 'space' for students to engage with clients in what seems a more passive manner at the outset can arguably better facilitate students' reflection on practice that Molloy and Keating identify as so important. Nonetheless, this unique approach embedded within a number of midwifery programmes resulted in instances where 'given their concern to be competent in their new practice, much of the student effort through the follow throughs was focused on procedural learning' (see Chapter 5, p. x, this volume).

As previously identified, the follow-through experiences were not directly facilitated, therefore, the active engagement of the students was very much self-directed with the effectiveness of the experience largely dependent on students' personal skills and abilities. Glover and Sweet (Chapter 5, this volume) acknowledge that the nature of this follow-through experience as presented is student-led, student-controlled and student-directed. In these ways, the follow-through experience therefore 'has the potential to greatly influence the development of agency in the student, and conversely, the agency of the student has the potential to greatly impact the learning outcomes of the follow through experience' (see Chapter 5, p. x, this volume).

In the ways outlined above, the design of the academic curriculum can directly contribute to shifting or reconfiguring priorities as perceived by students. Curriculum design can be instrumental in avoiding the problem of student-directed learning, as highlighted by Glover and Sweet (Chapter 5, this volume). Innovative approaches as presented in this book need to continue to be explored to further assist in the development of designs that broaden student professional learning. Specifically, designs that enhance professional abilities of engagement, interaction and reflection essential to deal with the complexity of human service and healthcare challenges are paramount. Human services (see Chapter 6, this volume) through a different nature of client interactions can potentially offer insights into developing students' ability to learn from practice experiences.

12.4 Structuring Learning Experiences to Promote Reflection in Practice

In addition to the actions aimed at positioning students within broad experiences are those direct interventions enacted for particular purposes. Staff engaged in human services need an expert repertoire of practices to even commence interactions with their clients, because these can be potentially confronting, difficult or even dangerous. Often the needs of these client groups are not so obvious as the needs of clients of other health services, for example, the woman giving birth (midwifery), the individual who has sustained muscular injury (physiotherapy) or the client physically recovering from a surgical procedure (nursing). The area of human services by its very nature (that is, the student is not readily able to focus on a physical ailment) has considerable challenges for students embarking on the clinical practicum. Cartmel (Chapter 6, this volume) identifies that it is essential for these students to have the confidence both personally and professionally when they engage with experiences. The difficulty is the preparation of these experiences – professional practice in the human services can be confronting and demanding, so there are significant challenges in preparing students for real-life scenarios.

While there are enormous challenges for adequate preparation of students, Cartmel (Chapter 6, this volume) introduces the notion that to better address these challenges it is necessary to engage the leaders and mentors in the practice arena. While this is not new – (see Newton et al., Chapter 3, this volume, whose interest was the preparation of the clinician to engage with the learner) – the powerful contribution of engaging with the providers in a 'learning circle approach' is that there is an equal dialogue and exchange of ideas across both parties, namely, academia and industry. Both industry and academia can add value to the experience of preparing the largely novice students to enter these environments.

Cartmel (Chapter 6, this volume) introduces Circles of Change (COC). Members of the COC comprise experienced practitioners, academics and students who contribute equally to exploring and contesting issues in practice. Diverse opinions about professional practice and multiple perspectives emerge from the conversations of the COCs. These experiences ideally contribute to the ability of the student to interact around, learn from and make sense of practice experiences. Students create new information about the abilities they need to be effective in their professional role. Ultimately, the COC approach provides participants with useful tools to enhance their ability to manage professional interactions. In particular, exploration and reflection upon experiences can assist in the development of resilience during field education when students join the workforce and need strategies to deal with confronting situations.

What emerges from the discussions in the chapters of this book is the need for careful consideration of the approach to the clinical practice experience, so that students can explore and be encouraged in the art of reflection to broaden their perspective and accommodate diverse understandings of the human condition. Enhancing students' ability, especially in the area of critical reflection, is particularly important in the work-integrated learning context because of the complexity of learning opportunities that arise. Discussion and reflection are essential practices in the working environment – and, therefore, it is important that they are effectively introduced to the students within the curricula and subsequently modelled by professionals.

12.5 The Contribution of Supervisors in Practice to Structure Student Learning

The contributions of more informed partners are likely to be necessary for effective learning in practice settings, because experiencing and participating alone are insufficient. In different ways, Newton et al. (Chapter 3, this volume), O'Keefe et al. (Chapter 11, this volume) and Henderson and Alexander (Chapter 8, this volume), through the accounts of student experiences in the real world, recognise the limitations of professionals' interactions to structure experiences for learning and facilitate students' engagement with practice that opens the students' lens to the learning opportunities. The concern introduced in these chapters is the notion that the practicing context, namely, the acute inpatient setting, aged-care or dental clinic, even across different professional groups is limited in its recognition of students, even those who may come equipped with advanced analytic and reflection skills. The realities of practice mean that these practicing clinicians may not necessarily be educated to shape learning opportunities or advance these students' capacities in understanding human and healthcare practice. The importance of the preparation of staff in contexts of practice became particularly evident across a range of areas.

Newton et al. (Chapter 3, this volume) identify a range of contemporary issues both outside of the control of the profession, for example, changes in demographics of the workforce, and those upon which the profession can make an impact, for example, cultures of practice (some of which do little to inspire reflective learning for students regardless of their preparation prior to entry to the clinical setting). These factors interact to configure the workplace learning experience for the student – namely, the level of engagement afforded to the student, the learning opportunities that the students seek and the situations at hand.

Consideration of both student preparation and the student placement within the community of practice is essential for enhancing the offerings of learning within practice. In the follow-through experience of midwifery, the students develop a rapport with the mother before becoming acquainted with the health professional and their domain of practice. Alternatively, in many of the other work-integrated experiences discussed in the chapters above, the students are introduced to the client through their association with the health professional who guides the student in the practice situation. The importance of effectively managing the placement within the community of practice is evident through the feedback from the midwifery follow-through experience: Students initially negotiated a 'social track' with the client as opposed to a professional track. This, in the longer term, created tension regarding the position of the student in relation to certain matters when interacting with the pregnant woman (see Chapter 5, this volume). Inclusion within the community of practice is essentially what work-integrated learning offers students – that is, the rich part of professionalism through which students observe, in which they participate and upon which they reflect. The challenge, therefore, arises in the curricula for students' preparation for the clinical experience to be consistent with the circumstances surrounding their placement within the community of practice. However, establishing the contingencies that best enable curricula objectives to be realised by students through the observations, learning and reflection from the experiences as they occur in the clinical contexts is not an exact science.

A productive engagement by staff and students within clinical settings is instrumental in creating an environment that invites new learners to become part of a team. The communities of practice, in which students find themselves situated, can be daunting. The students may not have been previously exposed to the situations they are now confronting. Indeed, work in healthcare inevitably places students in personally intimate situations in which clients are presented in revealing and novel ways that often elicit a barrage of emotions within novices. It is, therefore, important that the team has a commitment to guide student learning through the use of cues and clues that assists them draw on their academic studies. Newton et al. (Chapter 3, this volume) highlight essential characteristics of clinicians in practice, such as being competent and organised, supportive and motivating, and approachable with strong interpersonal skills, that can assist the student assimilate into the practice setting. When clinicians exhibit these skills, students are facilitated to become at ease with the real world of practice, including its unpredictable nature. Newton identifies that the social perspective offers insights to the expanse of cultural practices and products afforded to the individual in the workplace. When students are effectively guided by competent clinicians, a range of perspectives can ultimately provide rich learning experiences.

Diversity in understanding situations can be instrumental in shaping learning, and no more so than in the exemplar of interprofessional learning (see Chapter 8, this volume). Interprofessional learning is fraught with difficulties as it is not the core domain of any one profession. Consequently, support and guidance is not routinely given due attention across the domains of professional practice. In the way that it currently sits, support and guidance across professional groups is needed to support the learning of novices in the practice situation. Students need to be situated in the space and context where interprofessional practice is modelled appropriately, in order that they can learn the processes around this exemplary practice and replicate these in their own clinical work. Interprofessional learning in particular lends itself well to a work-integrated activity. The value of learning with other health professionals would be obvious to students if they recognised that such interaction would help them to learn more about the practice of providing healthcare. Exposure to interprofessional practice and effective guidance from health professionals around those factors that need to be considered for effective professional engagement is an important component of the learning that can aid smooth transitions for students upon graduation.

All of this emphasises the important role to be played by healthcare organisations' practices in shaping student learning.

12.6 Organisational Roles and Practices in Supporting Student Learning

As proposed by Henderson and Alexander (Chapter 8, this volume), there are many limitations to interprofessional learning. The first key factor is entrenched in students' perceptions and expectations. As identified earlier, these student perceptions are a major factor in shaping how and what students see as essential for professional practice and also what is important for 'getting through the programme,' often based in discipline-specific assessment tasks. As interprofessional learning is not routinely taught across the health disciplines, nor is assessment normally linked to any interprofessional learning activity, students normally do not view such opportunities for learning as important. If such learning is to be facilitated, then it is largely the practicing environment that needs to be instrumental in creating the opportunities for students to engage in interprofessional learning. A practical activity is presented by Henderson and Alexander, however, if this activity is not perceived as a relevant or worthwhile opportunity, that is, if it is not directly assessed as part of the clinical experience, then the development of interprofessional learning is reliant primarily on the context of care delivery. It is imperative that the community of practice is seen as an enabler of such activities that contribute to communication, teamwork and ideally collaboration that reaffirms to students the value of situational opportunities – a consistent feature of work-based learning. Without this perception, the basis by which learners engage is likely to be cautious and partial, with obvious consequences for their learning.

The importance and potential value of teams contributing to student learning is explored by O'Keefe et al. (Chapter 11, this volume). O'Keefe et al. recognise that health-service organisation, namely, teams and how they interact, significantly influences the ways in which students engage in their learning with the team members. While O'Keefe et al. recognise the importance of teams, they similarly recognise their potential to be very fluid in their composition. This fluidity is a constant phenomenon that is a result of teams needing to work rosters, the employment of part-time and casual staff, and the variable distribution of workloads (so that staff are shifted in and out of teams). O'Keefe et al. also recognise that the greater complexity of the health-service organisation, in terms of variability in clinical team composition, patient-care responsibilities and the overall size of the organisation, the fewer opportunities staff had to come together as a team to discuss student learning, namely appropriate placement, structuring of experiences and opportunities to engage in the dialogue around discussion of client needs. Two factors suggested to progress interprofessional learning are potentially relevant to also assisting the integration of teams to engage in student learning. Similar to many of the strategies examined by O'Keefe et al. (Chapter 11, this volume), these initiatives largely sit outside the existing curriculum. They are based in principles that acknowledge the need for good communication and understanding across academia and industry. Momentum for learning that is to accommodate the complexities of contemporary practice, for example, interprofessional work, variable team membership and representation, and diverse client groups and needs, is best enabled through effective leadership across academia and industry and true engagement between these two parties (Creedy & Henderson, 2009).

- Leadership: Senior leaders need to recognise the extent of their influence on practice and the values inherent in that practice. Curriculum needs to introduce students to the situational factors that can influence practice and learning. Leadership is instrumental in establishing the organisation's priorities and what is valued – accordingly dialogue and sharing is needed across both academic and industry partners to ensure alignment and understanding of the student learning in these contexts. Communication that enhances student inquiry and learning is powerful in shaping the context where students feel readily invited to participate in and engage with the community.
- Engagement by stakeholders, namely, clinicians: Clinicians, as recognised by both Newton et al. (Chapter 3, this volume) and O'Keefe et al. (Chapter 11, this volume), are fundamental to student learning. And as O'Keefe et al. duly recognise – just as clinicians are the basis of students' technical learning, how clinicians interact within a team is just as significant for student learning about communication, collaboration and teamwork. Ideally, these existing communication mechanisms within the group that are used to discuss clinical matters impact on communication around student learning. When these mechanisms work effectively, they can similarly be used to assist with student feedback and the opportunity for students to reflect on their learning experiences. O'Keefe et al. identify that, possibly because of the clearly circumscribed dental team, every member of the team knew about the student's placement and learning objectives, even though they may not have been directly supervising the dental students' practice.

Leadership that supports learning in clinical practice environments, engagement of clinicians to teach and interact with students and the identification of relevant activities in which students may engage during the clinical experience are important considerations for the affordances that the students are offered. The challenge for the academic sector relates to how to establish the operation of these essential facets that engage work-based teams within the parameters of the curricula so that organisations that are seemingly peripheral to student learning become an investment by the tertiary sector to enable student-learning opportunities. As recognised by Newton et al. (Chapter 3, this volume), it is essential that clinicians are aware of student-learning needs and how best to interact with students. Furthermore, the recognition of the complexity of teams is essential if universities are to better understand how to interact with these work-based settings so that students do not merely participate in one-on-one interactions but, rather, are afforded optimum learning experiences through their inclusion in highly effective teams that not just organise and plan the experiences but also facilitate opportunities where the team learns from each other and students can benefit through participation in this learning. There are many factors not the least of which are heavy workloads and the focus on the delivery of a clinical service as quite clearly explained by O'Keefe et al. (Chapter 11, this volume) that serve to counteract attempts by the academic sector to engage clinicians in dialogue about the facilitation of student learning. The chapters through the course of the book have unearthed a myriad of tensions and challenges – for all parties from the student, to the clinician with whom they work to the team that comprises the community of learning where the student is situated.

12.7 Expanding Possibilities for Workplace Learning

For students to engage in professional activities, that is, to be adequately sequenced and guided through practice via the subtle cues of health professionals, students need to be well positioned in a practice community. Ideally, within this practice community, dialogue and sharing between the members, whether the community is comprised of practitioners, students and academics, or whether it is comprised of health practitioners and students, is routinely demonstrated and modelled. These activities when embedded within practice can facilitate critical reflection on practice, essential if students are to make sense of their academic knowledge and practice, and also if they are to continue their learning and development as a professional subsequent to their initial registration or qualification.

Strategies for professional growth through active engagement with learning opportunities are a key feature and need to be well structured within the curriculum (and ultimately necessitate greater interaction with clinical settings). Many studies identify that there are gaps between curricular intentions and students' experience. They suggest that educators need to model reflective practice. Critical reflection needs to be considered as 'core' business, and accordingly educators need to create a curriculum that situates critical reflection in this way. While this is fundamental, it also needs to be modelled not just in the educational institution but also in the workplace. Drawing on a similar use of reflective practice was also advocated by Glover and Sweet (Chapter 5, this volume) in the very independent work that the student lives during the follow-through experience. They suggest that reflective practice is essential to capture and enrich learning. Midwifery students need to be prepared to reflect on practice and therefore require assistance with understanding the difference between description and reflection and how best to use these for learning.

The context of practice is important in structuring students' exposure to complex situations in order that students can learn the essential techniques of practice but also have the opportunity to discuss and share their observations in order to derive meaning from their experiences. An imperative component of this is how professionals interact and structure and guide student learning within these situations. The contexts of the practice communities as presented in the work of Newton et al. (Chapter 3, this volume), Newton (Chapter 7, this volume), O'Keefe et al. (Chapter 11, this volume) and Henderson and Alexander (Chapter 8, this volume) present many circumstances that arise in workplace learning, and ultimately make enormous impacts on student learning. Unfortunately, the potencies of organisational practices' impacts are presently not a major consideration for the university nor are they given serious consideration as a pivotal component of curriculum activity that can make an enormous contribution to the optimal functioning of these students upon graduation.

Aligning curricula with the professional skills and abilities necessary for beginning level practitioners is essential if students are to continue their learning and growth upon their initial registration. It is imperative that processes integral to WIL create the context so that appropriate learning activities are sufficiently sequenced in practice to ensure their optimal development in the student. Positive partnerships between the academic institution and the clinical settings where students are situated within practice communities are needed to assist clinicians to guide and sequence learning opportunities for students within the complexities of real practice.

12.8 Summary

Learning that guides students around the practice of the application of skills, knowledge and abilities with work contexts is fraught with tensions. These tensions can emerge initially from a lack of alignment of the students' expectations and the intent of the curricula and can be further compounded by the realities of practice settings that are not clearly prepared to role-model and guide professional learning, and this lack of preparation also means that learning does not arise sequentially.

Constraining factors around optimal affordances for students in human and health-service agencies pertain to students' preconceived notions of their learning that can contribute to other opportunities being 'missed'; limited invitations to engage and limitations in the extent of engagement that can result in hesitancy by students to interact – and this can result in an approach whereby they 'do not rock the boat.'

Key considerations for the appropriate preparation of students so that they can maximise affordances include preparation strategies for students to assist them manage the immediacy of learning situations, increased engagement of clinicians with students to structure and guide their learning, and the use of facilitation strategies that promote dialogue and reflection with the student to maximise learning.

The success of these initiatives is dependent on engagement across academia and practice-based settings that assist both students and staff in the requisites of learning and strategies through which these can be achieved. Deliberate learning structured by clinicians ideally addresses the contextual and emergent factors surrounding healthcare that are so important in equipping graduates for contingencies of contemporary practice. Practices need to be organised so that students think and reflect as opposed to perform routine tasks in order to develop problem-solving and decision-making skills necessary to deliver sound professional judgement.

Acknowledgements The author wishes to acknowledge the support provided by the Australian Learning and Teaching Council.

References

Brammer, J. (2006). A phenomenographic study of registered nurses' understanding of their role in student learning – An Australian perspective. *International Journal of Nursing Studies, 43*, 963–973.

Creedy, D., & Henderson, A. (2009). *Leading for effective partnering in clinical contexts*. Retrieved December 26, 2009, from <http://www.altc.edu.au/project-leading-effective-partnering-griffith-2006>

Ericson, K. A. (2006). The influence of experience and deliberate practice on the development of superior expert performance. In K. A. Ericsson, N. Charness, P. J. Feltowich, & R. R. Hoffmann (Eds.), *The Cambridge handbook of expertise and expert performance* (pp. 685–705). Cambridge: Cambridge University Press.

Joint Quality Initiative informal group. (2004). *Complete set Dublin Descriptors 2004 1.31.doc*. Retrieved August 18, 2010, from http://www.jointquality.nl/

Rodger, S., Webb, G., Devitt, L., Gilbert, J., Wrightson, P., & McMeeken, J. (2008). Clinical education and practice placements in the allied health professions: An international perspective. *Journal of Allied Health, 37*(1), 53–62.

Name Index

S. Billett, A. Henderson (eds.), *Developing Learning Professionals*, Professional
and Practice-based Learning 7, DOI 10.1007/978-90-481-3937-8,
© Springer Science+Business Media B.V. 2011

Subject Index

CPSIA information can be obtained at www.ICGtesting.com
Printed in the USA
LVOW01*1924080415

433784LV00006B/59/P